The Acid Alkaline Balance Diet

REVISED EDITION

An Innovative Program That Detoxifies
Your Body's Acidic Waste to Prevent Disease
and Restore Overall Health

Felicia Drury Kliment

New York Chicago San Francisco Lisbon London Madrid Mexico City
Milan New Delhi San Juan Seoul Singapore Sydney Toronto

The *McGraw·Hill* Companies

Library of Congress Cataloging-in-Publication Data

Kliment, Felicia Drury.
    The acid-alkaline balance diet : an innovative program that detoxifies your
body's acidic waste to prevent disease and restore overall health / by Felicia Drury Kliment.
—[2nd ed.].
            p.   cm.
    Includes bibliographical references and index.
    ISBN-13: 978-0-07-170337-6
    ISBN-10: 0-07-170337-3
    1. Acid-base imbalances—Diet therapy.   2. Acid-base imbalances—Complications.
    I. Title.

    RC630.K565   2010
    616.3'992—dc22   2009043029

To Stephen
Always with us

2 3 4 5 6 7 8 9 10 11 12 13 14 15 16 17 18 19   WFR/WFR   1 9 8 7 6 5 4 3 2 1 0

ISBN 978-0-07-170337-6
MHID   0-07-170337-3

The information in this book is not intended to be a substitute for the medical advice of
physicians. The reader should consult his or her doctor in all matters relating to health.
Although every effort has been made to ensure that information is presented accurately in this
book, the ultimate responsibility for proper medical treatment rests with the physician. Neither
the author nor the publisher can be held responsible for errors or for any consequences arising
from the use of information contained here.

CONTENTS

ACKNOWLEDGMENTS

Fiona Sarne, my editor, has the rare ability to see the large picture and at the same time never miss a detail. Her advice is always on target, and she is a pleasure to work with. Thanks to Susan Moore for her attention to detail and thoroughness in seeing the book through production. Also, thanks to my daughter, Pamela, and my son-in-law, Steve, for their invaluable advice and wisdom.

INTRODUCTION

A Personal Odyssey

It took me twenty years of researching, writing, and consulting in the field of alternative health before I found the common denominator in all degenerative disease: acidic waste. These wastes are largely the by-products of the food we eat. Wherever acid waste accumulates, it causes nearby organs to malfunction and degenerate.

Before I ever became aware that acidic wastes could cause serious health problems, I was unknowingly devising simple strategies to reduce the toxic acid levels in my body. After a stressful day at work, I would take a hot bath—unusual for me, as I am a confirmed shower taker—or drink some hot milk. I later learned that hot baths and hot milk reduce excess acidity in the urine, and this has a calming effect on the nerves. A remedy I used for an upset stomach was an ice pack. It gave me relief within seconds. I read later in the medical journal *Lancet* that cold temperatures stimulate the production of antihistamines—as the name implies, they destroy histamines, which are the cause of allergic reactions.

Yet if you had asked me at the time if elevated acid levels were dangerous to health, I would have denied it. Despite being knowledgeable about the physiology of the body, I knew nothing about hyperacidity. After all, my mother had had acid indigestion all her life, and she died at the age of ninety-eight, still able to live by herself. Whenever she had a stomach upset, she used an old folk remedy handed down from her mother: one-eighth teaspoon each of bicarbonate of soda, spirits of ammonia, and essence of peppermint. The alkalinity of the ammonia, bicarbonate of soda, and peppermint neutralized the acidic residues in her stomach—the by-products of foods not adequately broken down.

While I was successfully (if unknowingly) treating my own symptoms of acidity, those who had come to me for advice on how to alleviate their health problems were not all so lucky. Some felt no better after they had taken my advice than before. An abundance of health foods, herbs, and vitamins had passed through their bodies and had no effect. Something was missing.

A Chinese acupuncturist friend gave me a clue. Aware of the ancient Chinese belief that all living and nonliving things were predominantly yin or yang, I asked her what these opposites actually meant. She answered, "Yin is acid; yang is alkaline." This was exactly what I had learned in chemistry, namely, that all earthly elements were made up of different combinations of acid particles (positively charged protons) and alkaline particles (negatively charged electrons). It is the magnetic attractions and repulsions between these particles that cause atoms to form molecules, molecular chains, and ionic compounds, the building blocks of the body's tissues and fluids. It follows that normal body function depends on the correct balance of acid and alkaline particles in the blood, lymph, enzymes, urine, and other body fluids. This was the factor that I had overlooked in the health problems of my patients.

I knew that the Chinese treated illness by using yin and yang herbs and acupuncture needles to bring about a balance in the body between these two opposing principles. I had a hunch that I could get even better results in restoring acid-alkaline balance in the body using diet and alkaline particles to rid the body of acidic wastes.

While acid and alkaline substances are both vital to life, acid favors the decomposition of living things, while alkaline (or base) prevents it. Examples of this are the corpses buried in the fourteenth century under the cathedral of Venzone in Italy. Some corpses have remained intact, while others have become skeletons. The dead bodies interred where the underground water contains a high concentration of alkaline-forming lime have become mummified, whereas the flesh of the bodies buried in places where the water is highly acidic has been eaten away by bacteria.[1]

Once I came to understand the destruction that elevated acid waste levels in the body could cause, I made their removal my first priority in restoring health. The client of mine who perhaps benefited most from my new approach was José, born in Peru and now living in New York with his family. He was sixteen when he began having pains in his abdomen. The doctors couldn't decide whether the pain came from an infected appendix or stones in the gallbladder, so to "play it safe," they had both organs surgically removed. Shortly after, José developed systemic lupus erythematosus (SLE), usually referred to as lupus, an autoimmune disease in which the internal organs are destroyed by the body's own immune system. The disease used to be fatal, usually within three years of onset. Now a combination of prednisone and chemotherapy keeps patients alive for a considerable period of time—unless the immune system is strong enough to overcome the toxicity of the chemotherapy and attacks the kidneys, which was the case with José.

José's immune cells had eaten holes in his kidneys. As a result, his kidneys leaked protein, which pooled in the lower part of the body and in the urine, causing his ankles and feet to swell and turning his urine brown. José had lost fifty pounds. Because it was obvious to his mother that he was losing his battle to stay alive, she asked me for help.

Although José had given up all soft drinks on orders from his doctor, his lupus indicated that he was suffering the aftereffects of having drunk six to eight bottles of cola a day, starting at the age of seven. Soft drinks, particularly colas, are said to be so acidic that José would have had to drink thirty-two glasses of water to neutralize a single glass of Coke! I suggested to José that he drink five glasses daily of an alkaline juice made from bitter and bland-tasting vegetables such as celery, spinach, bitter melon, lettuce, and zucchini squash to clear out the acidic wastes that had to have accumulated in his body from his soft drink addiction.

After only one week on this juice regimen, José began to show slight signs of improvement. Since the Coumadin (a drug also used as a rat poison) that the doctor had prescribed for a large blood clot in his leg had not dissolved the clot, I had José start taking 200 units of vitamin E a day, gradually increasing the dose to 1,600 units.

Three weeks after he started to take vitamin E, José's kidneys stopped leaking, the swelling in his feet and ankles was down, and his blood clot disappeared. José's lupus is now in remission.

José was the first of many individuals I advised who regained their health after the acid waste that was causing their illness was removed from their body. The successful outcome of this treatment in the vast majority of cases has led me to believe that the removal of acidic wastes should be the first factor in restoring health.

Balancing acid-alkaline pH and preventing degenerative disease is possible under only one condition—when you have enough of the right kind of digestive enzymes to break down the food you eat, so there are no leftover food particles that turn toxic by acidifying.

The solution is to include in your diet only those foods that your digestive enzymes can handle. To find out what these foods are, take the Metabolic-Type Niacin Test (see Chapter 2). The results reveal whether your digestive requirements fit that of a meat eater, which means that you have too much stomach acid; a grain, fish, and fowl eater, a sign of too little stomach acid; or a balanced metabolism (you have normal quantities of acids and other kinds of digestive enzymes and therefore can handle all kinds of protein). As you'll see later on when we look at specific diseases in relation to acidic waste, eating based on your metabolic type is critical to preventing disease and restoring overall health.

The Health Benefits of a Metabolically Appropriate Diet

The most obvious benefit from eating foods that are digested well is a greater supply of food molecules available to the cells for carrying out their intracellular functions. Well-digested food also means fewer left-over food molecules that turn into acid waste. When acid waste in the blood is reduced, elevated stress hormone levels, such as estrogen and cortisol, return to normal and we feel calmer. Lowering acid waste also helps balance organ function. When all the organs are functioning at the same speed, healing is accelerated. Lowered acid waste levels provide other benefits as well. By keeping estrogen levels low—men also have estrogen, only in smaller quantities than women—oxygen is preserved. Disease prevention depends on this because oxygen destroys cancer cells and is essential to the cells' production of energy.

Perhaps most important of all, when acid waste levels have decreased to the point where the only acidic waste in the body is from normal cellular function, organs don't become inflamed and degenerate.

Part I of *The Acid-Alkaline Balance Diet* deals with the dangers of acid waste from undigested food and explains the different ways you can detoxify your body—whether the toxicity consists of acidified food debris, heavy metals, or man-made chemicals. It also reveals how you can prevent autoimmune disease.

In Part II, each chapter is devoted to a particular health problem and contains newly discovered nutritional supplements and foods that have a healing effect. There are also dozens of heartrending stories about individuals, who, by following the advice recounted in these chapters, have escaped a life of chronic illness and, in some cases, death.

ACIDIC WASTES: THE REAL CULPRIT BEHIND DEGENERATIVE DISEASE AND AUTOIMMUNE DISORDERS

CHAPTER 1

HOW ACIDIC WASTES CAUSE DISEASE

Detoxification is even more important to longevity than good nutrition. French physiologist Alexia Carrell kept pieces of chicken heart tissue alive in a solution containing the same mineral levels found in chicken blood plasma for twenty-eight years.[1] The cells in the tissue stopped dividing and died out only when he stopped changing the solution, although he continued to place minerals in the solution in the same amount. The chicken heart cells, despite being provided with the necessary nutrients, could not carry on their metabolic activities because the fluid in which they were placed had become filled with acid wastes.

The environment of the human body cannot be so easily purified as the test-tube environment of Carrell's chicken heart tissue. The body's detoxifying organs—liver, lymph, immune system, kidneys, and lungs—were not designed to neutralize synthetic chemicals and heavy metal contaminants that have found their way into the body in recent years.

The hydrogenation of edible oils leaves behind traces of aluminum and nickel, and food additives contain remnants of such toxic heavy metals as cadmium, lead, mercury, and chromium. Mercury from dental amalgams and in canned tuna fish, the formaldehyde and mercury in vaccines, and the lead from car exhaust are just a few of the multitudes of toxins that have found their way into the body.[2]

The chemist Ray Peat, Ph.D., writes, "Heavy metals accumulate in the body at a faster rate as the body ages, and have an affinity for the bones. Lead, in particular, replaces bone calcium. And heavy metals can trigger the onset of bone cancer by replacing the blood-making machinery in the bones. Some materials such as chelators and EDTA (a mild acid used in chelation) move metals from the bones to the brain where they are more destructive."[3]

Fortunately there are ways we can help the body reduce its store of heavy metals and synthetic chemicals. A juice made with vegetables high in alkaline minerals such as celery and parsley can neutralize heavy metals in the lungs. Lemon juice in water before breakfast is an effective detoxifier of heavy metals in general. With its heavy concentration of negatively charged ions, the lemon in the water bonds with positively charged metal molecules and neutralizes them. Once neutralized, the body has no problem eliminating them.

Mineral supplements are also helpful in reducing heavy metals. Calcium, iron, and copper lower lead levels; vitamin C, zinc, and selenium remove mercury from the body; and zinc, copper, and iron reduce cadmium levels.

The body has another means of eliminating some of the potent acids that leach out of pesticides, heavy metals, and food debris and settle in the blood. But this system does not eliminate them. It just gets them out of harm's way. When the body's slightly alkaline blood pH is threatened by the acidity of these foreign intruders, the body binds them with

ANN LOSES WEIGHT AFTER SHE GIVES UP HORMONE-FED BEEF

Avoiding foods that contain additives can yield health benefits. Ann, a client of mine, was addicted to meat when she lived in the United States, but when she moved to Mexico where the cattle's only source of food is grass, she lost her craving. Ann had weighed 30 pounds more when she ate meat from hormone-fed, U.S.-raised steer than she does now on a diet of hormone-free beef. Her experience is an example of the accelerating effect of hormones on appetite, and the increase in weight that results from it.

calcium, an alkaline mineral, and deposits them as far away as possible from the circulating blood.[4]

As we age, the wastes in our bodies accumulate in such great quantities that the body is unable to dispose of them, so they calcify. By the time most people reach the age of fifty, they have acquired a few enlarged knuckles, calcium spurs in the heel, and calcified deposits on the vertebrae and in muscle tissue. These calcium deposits can be painful but are not life-threatening.

Acidity and Cardiovascular Disease

Acidic wastes are not always rendered less harmful by being safely entombed in calcium deposits. When the body's acidic load becomes too large, some acid particles remain in the blood. They trigger the onset of cardiovascular disease by making scratches and bumps on the inside walls of arteries. These injuries are "bandaged" over with cholesterol, triglycerides, calcium, and other wastes. Of course, the higher the cholesterol and triglyceride levels, the thicker the "bandage" and the narrower the arteries.

A high cholesterol level is not the underlying cause of hardening of the arteries. Cholesterol and other thick, sticky substances cannot adhere to vessel walls that are smooth. Only after the arterial vessel walls become pitted and scratched by acid particles are fatty plaques able to stick to them.

Narrowed arteries are dangerous for two reasons. Fatty plaques are more likely to become detached from vessel walls and trigger the formation of blood clots, which travel through the bloodstream to the brain and cause strokes. They also raise blood pressure, increasing the likelihood of heart attacks and strokes.

That the injury of arterial walls by acid particles is the major cause of high blood pressure is strongly indicated by the clinical studies of Dr. Kancho Kuninaha, who successfully lowered the blood pressure of many of his patients with alkaline water.[5] Normalized blood pressure readings indicated that the arteries had opened up, and the alkaline particles in the water had removed the fatty plaques and acidic wastes from the arterial walls.

Acidity, Autoimmune Disorders, and Food Allergies

The groundwork is laid for autoimmune disease when the immune cells decide a particular food is an unfriendly microbe. To "protect" the body from this "enemy," the immune cells not only trigger the production of histamines but also maneuver an enzyme into making a leak in the intestines. Those food molecules the immune cells have designated as hostile, not knowing what the immune system is up to, slip through these leaks. Once in the general circulation they become sitting ducks for the immune cells. The latter, however, in the process of disposing of the food allergens, become inflamed and mutate. In their new guise the immune cells attack the body's own protoplasm. Proof that it is not uncommon for the immune system to be transformed from a "Dr. Jekyll" to a "Mr. Hyde" is the fact that there are now sixty-three clinically proven autoimmune disorders, including celiac disease, lupus, rheumatoid arthritis and osteoarthritis, type 1 diabetes, and Crohn's disease.

To prevent autoimmune disease, avoid eating foods that you know you are allergic to. If you are not sure what these foods are, test yourself (see the Pulse Test in Chapter 2). Also, keep in mind that any symptoms, no matter how removed they seem from those caused by food allergies, may nevertheless be due to them. The most common reactions caused by histamines are rashes, eczema, swelling, insomnia, headaches, drowsiness, dizziness, arthritic pain, and sleeplessness.

Acidity and Cancer

While the health of the cardiovascular system is threatened most by injuries inflicted by acid particles in arteries, the other organs of the body—the liver, pancreas, lungs, and so on—are more likely to degenerate when acidic wastes accumulate in the nearby capillaries that feed them. Acid wastes thicken the blood, and the coagulated blood cannot carry the quantity of nutrients and oxygen the organs need to function efficiently.

When we refer to the malfunction of organs, we really mean the abnormal function of the millions of cells that make up each organ. These cells depend on, among other things, oxygen to manufacture energy and amino acids for the synthesis of protein and the division of old cells into new ones. When the cell is deprived of these substances, it either dies or adapts to the new oxygen-deprived environment by becoming malignant. The cancer cell can live in such an environment for two reasons. First, it obtains its energy from fermentation, a process that is carried on without oxygen. Second, multiplying continually, it grabs the nutrients designated for the body's normal cells. The latter, deprived of their sustenance, are either gobbled up by the rapidly multiplying cancer cells or they stop dividing and die.

Clearly, the prevention of cancer should begin with removing from the body acidic wastes that turn normal cells into cancerous ones. If an individual is being treated for cancer, the removal of acidic wastes generated by chemotherapy could prevent a recurrence.

My friend Maureen and I were having lunch together for the first time in three years. I was struck by how healthy and youthful she looked at the age of sixty-five. I asked her to what she attributed her survival from breast cancer surgery some fifteen years before, even though she had been told after the mastectomy of her left breast that her cancer had spread to her lymph glands. She answered, "During the five years I was on tamoxifen, I never took an antinausea pill. Instead, I let myself throw up whenever I needed to." In doing this, Maureen had deprived her cancer cells of the acidic environment in which they thrive.

Acidity and Alcoholism

On the surface, there does not seem to be a connection between cancer and alcoholism—yet the purging of acidic wastes is effective in both cases. In his book *A Monk Swimming: A Memoir*,[6] Malachy McCourt wrote that at the age of seventy-two, after a lifetime of nightly intoxication, he was still healthy thanks to the fact that he "knelt down in the bathroom" after he came home from his nightly binges. By throwing up the acids generated in his digestive tract by the alcohol, McCourt spared his liver the damage it would have sustained from acid aldehyde, the highly toxic by-product of alcohol.

CHAPTER 2

RIDDING YOUR BODY
OF ACIDIC WASTES

Twenty-five years ago, my husband and I spent a week on the island of Nevis, known to its inhabitants as "the pearl of the Caribbean." It was at that time entirely unspoiled. Hiking along a coastal road that circled the island, we came across a village woman said to be 106 years old. She sat in front of the open door of her hut; before her was a grill. A bubbling sound came from a big frying pan placed on top of it in which she was boiling soft-shell crabs. These crabs and the other seafood she ate daily came directly from the ocean no more than fifty yards from her hut. The rest of her food supplies were even closer at hand. As we looked around at the sloping sides of the valley in which her hut was situated, we noticed rows of squash and other vegetables wedged between tangles of tropical foliage.

The key to her longevity, we suspected, was that she lived her life in accordance with the cycles of nature. The nutrient loss in the foods she ate was minimal, since the fish and plants were alive only minutes before she prepared and ate them. She got her seafood from the fishermen just returned from their early-morning fishing expeditions, as they tied their boats to the dock. By raising vegetables in her own "backyard," she satisfied two basic tenets of good health: she ate food that was locally grown and what was in season. Since the tropical weather enabled her to grow her vegetable garden all year long, she never had to resort to canned or frozen food, thus avoiding the chemical preservatives and nutrient loss characteristic of processed food.

The chance encounter with this ancient but vigorous lady and her organically grown garden in the midst of natural surroundings illustrates the benefits to health achieved by following one's traditional diet and of eating foods plucked fresh from earth and sea. It also points up the contrast to our own lives, which have been damaged by modern agriculture and food preservation methods, as well as a scientific theory that doesn't take into account the detrimental effects of processing and chemical additives in assessing the nutritional value of food.

Acidic and Alkaline Foods—Achieving a Balance

Dr. R. A. Wiley, a physicist, described in his book *Bio Balance* six diets for individuals with mental disorders. Wiley assigned these diets to the subjects in his study according to their acid-alkaline blood pH.[1] There are several reasons why this diet can't work.

First, there is a difference of opinion as to which foods are acid forming and which alkaline forming. For example, bananas, avocados, asparagus, artichokes, and spinach are considered by Zen Buddhists to be acid producing, while Western scientists believe them to be alkaline because, when burned, they leave behind more alkaline mineral ashes than acidic ones.

Furthermore, many acid-forming vegetables that nutritionists involved in balancing pH tell us to eat less of are nevertheless very effective in eliminating acidic waste. The juice of carrots and beets, with their high percentage of acid-forming minerals—sulfur and phosphorus—effectively clean out the acidic wastes from the liver, kidneys, and bladder. The juice of cabbage, high in acid-forming chlorine and sulfur, cleanses the acid wastes adhering to the mucous membranes of the stomach and intestinal tract. An excellent remedy for gum disease and infections in general is the highly acidic vitamin C.

Alkaline minerals are also effective cleansers. Potassium, calcium, sodium, and magnesium in dandelions, endive, and lettuce reduce hyperacidity in all the organs. Indeed, acid and alkaline minerals act together to cleanse the body, just as a combined solution of vinegar (acid) and bicarbonate of soda (alkaline) makes an excellent household cleaner.

The Difference Between Acidic Waste and Acidic Foods

Acidic waste and acidic foods have opposite effects on the body. Acid waste is destructive—it eats up oxygen and inflames tissue. Sour-tasting (acidic) foods, on the other hand, supply the body with the acid it needs to digest protein.

Proof that acidic food staples do not threaten the blood's pH factor or cause degenerative disease are the several populations that have what the "experts" claim are predominantly acidic diets. Yet they are known for their longevity. One example is the macrobiotic diet developed by Dr. Sagen Ishizuka in the latter half of the nineteenth century to cure his kidney disease, which Western medicine had failed to do. Although it is based on the concept of balancing opposites—yin (acid) and yang (alkaline)—the dietary staple of the macrobiotic diet is brown rice, which contains a high level of acid-forming phosphorus.

Dr. Weston Price, an American dentist, traveled during the 1930s in Africa, the outback of Australia, and the Arctic to study the relationship between diet and health in the tribes in these regions, which still followed the traditional diets of their forefathers.[2] He found that many of the tribes who followed a grain-based diet, which is high in acid-forming phosphorous, were in robust health, free of cardiovascular disease and cancer.

It seems that a diet high in alkaline minerals is not necessary either for the maintenance of health or for a normal 7.4 alkaline pH blood plasma. Normalizing acid-alkaline blood pH by eating more foods higher in alkaline-forming minerals than acidic ones should not be the basis for working out a diet for two more reasons: First, clusters of acidic, toxic wastes in various parts of the body don't necessarily raise blood acid levels. It is doubtful that balancing the blood pH through diet would make any inroads into concentrations of acidic wastes located far from major blood supplies. Second, the amount of enzymes, bile, hydrochloric acid, and other metabolites the body manufactures for the breakdown of nutrients is not determined by the blood pH but by the particular food flavors and protein that sustained the individual's ancestors for thousands of years.

A Young Girl Benefits from Following Her Ancestral Diet

Dawanta was born with sickle-cell anemia. When I met her she was seventeen years old and getting four pints of blood every month. Her sickle-cell gene was an inheritance from her ancestors who lived in the equatorial region of Africa. Ironically, the sickle-cell gene in Africa is beneficial because it prevents malaria—rampant along the equator because of the infection-carrying mosquitoes that proliferate in this swampy region. Despite the prevalence of the sickle-cell gene in Africans living near the equator, it was rare that anyone came down with the disease. What prevented the gene's expression was the dietary staple of the Africans: the cassava root.

Being aware of these facts, I recommended to Dawanta's grandmother that she make cassava for Dawanta once a day, and to make it according to the traditional African recipe. (Peel the barklike skin, grate it raw, and cook it in a little water until the mucilage is released and the cassava achieves a gluelike texture.) After one month on the cassava, Dawanta was able to stretch the time between blood transfusions from one month to two months and to cut down on her blood transfusions from four pints to two. Given the healing effect of cassava on Dawanta's sickle-shaped red blood cells even though she was already in her teens, imagine what cassava could have done for her had it been a regular part of her diet from the time she was a baby.

Dawanta's story points up the advantage to health of continuing the dietary traditions of one's ancestors, particularly of their dietary staple. If your ancestors were primarily meat eaters you should make meat the staple of your diet. If your ancestors had a diet heavy in fish, you should eat fish two or three times a week. On the other hand, individuals of Asian descent benefit from following the grain-eating traditions of their cultures. The fact is that nutrients not part of a person's cultural heritage are incompatible with that individual's biochemistry. Solomon Katz of the University of Pennsylvania has proven in his research that people's genetic makeup is shaped by their food practices.[3] A case in point are those U.S. immigrants from India who have replaced their grain diet with meat. They have experienced a sharp increase in heart disease.

Not all individuals, however, have the same metabolism as their ancestors. Most people in the United States are of mixed descent, and there are variations in individual metabolisms within any given population cluster. A simple, self-administered test (explained later in this chapter) can determine whether you have a grain-eating or meat-eating metabolism or whether your digestive apparatus can handle all kinds of protein.

During the earlier part of the twentieth century in the United States, the general public viewed health in relation to nutrition either in terms of providing food for the hungry or, for those who had enough to eat, the balanced meal. This was a meal in which the three food groups— protein, carbohydrates, and fats—were well represented. Textbooks typically described food according to food type, weight in grams, and calories. The implication was that the processing of foods and chemical additives did not affect nutritional quality. In the 1960s on the office wall of my children's pediatrician was a poster featuring the ideal dinner—a plate containing a lamb chop, mashed potatoes with butter, some corn (canned), a slice of white bread with a pat of butter, a glass of milk, and canned fruit and a cookie for dessert.

The sacred aura surrounding the balanced meal dimmed somewhat when mainstream medicine began to take notice of statistical research studies done in the 1950s. These studies showed that during World War II, Europeans, deprived of butter and fatty meat, did not develop cardiovascular disease to the extent that they did before the war. In fact, subsequent studies revealed they died of such infectious diseases as tuberculosis before they were old enough to develop hardened arteries. A healthy diet was now considered to be one in which polyunsaturated oils replaced animal and dairy fats—even though studies have long linked polyunsaturates with cancer.

By the 1980s the medical establishment began advocating fruits and vegetables because studies showed they prevented degenerative disease. The research studies were undertaken largely in response to the public's interest in the subject and the growing market for organically grown produce and whole grains.

While Dr. Weston Price equated good health with natural foods such as raw milk and butter, fresh produce, and whole-grain flour, Dr. Roger J. Williams, a biochemist who did his research studies in the middle of the twentieth century, viewed nutrition in terms of the nutrients that make up food: amino acids, fatty acids, starch, vitamins, and minerals. But breaking up food into its component parts is the only similarity between Williams and the mainstream medical establishment at that time. Williams was revolutionary in his assertions that cellular malnutrition, rather than bacteria and viruses, was the major cause of disease. He backed up his theory with his research on yeast cells, which showed that the efficiency with which a cell carried out its metabolic activities is determined by the nourishment it receives.[4] He found further that cells die off not only because they don't get everything they need but also because they are poisoned by chemical additives.

Williams not only brought to light the error in the thinking of doctors and nutritionists that good nutrition as a disease preventative meant eating adequate amounts of protein, carbohydrates, fats, and sugar without regard to vitamin and mineral content; he also pointed at individual differences in the size and shape of organs, even the microscopic organs (organelles) within the cell. He concluded that these structural differences were inherited, and along with diet they had a profound effect on physical and mental health. Williams, then, recognized two biological truths that continue to be given short shrift by the medical establishment: the needs of the body's metabolic machinery for quantities of vitamins, minerals, and amino acids that cannot be obtained from processed foods, and the connection between variability in organ structure and function and the individual's state of health. He also came to the conclusion that individuals who are susceptible to disease have, because of their biochemical individuality, distinctive patterns of nutritional needs.

Williams, however, did not explore this issue further. He simply hypothesized that the nutritional requirements of individuals were determined by either susceptibility or resistance to disease. When Williams conducted his research (from the 1930s through the 1960s), little information was available on individual differences in metabolism and how they determine dietary requirements. As a result Williams viewed diet only from the perspective of disease prevention and treatment. For example, he recommended the I. M. Stillman diet for anyone who was overweight (lean meat, poultry, fish, seafood, cottage cheese, low dessert, and almost no carbohydrates and fat) without regard to individual differences in body structure and biochemistry.

Dr. Max Gerson, an immigrant from Nazi Germany, used diet and detoxification in the 1940s and 1950s to heal advanced cancers. In his book *A Cancer Therapy*, Gerson described fifty "terminal" cancer cases that he cured.[5] Like Williams, he recommended a single diet for the cure and prevention of illness. He stated that 75 percent of the diet should consist of fresh raw, juiced, or stewed fruits and vegetables that "contain all the necessary nutritional substances in their proper quantity, mixture, and composition."

In the 1970s Dr. William Donald Kelley, a dentist and nutritionist, was one of the first health-care professionals to recognize that individual variation in autonomic nervous system function created different food metabolisms. The nerves of the autonomic nervous system are composed of two branches, the parasympathetic and sympathetic, each regulating a different set of organ systems. The parasympathetic nerves ensure the survival of the internal body environment by accelerating the processes of digestion and assimilation of food, elimination of waste products, and repair and rebuilding of body cells. The sympathetic nerves, on the other hand, protect the body from the environment outside the body by speeding up the flow of hormones from the thyroid, adrenals, and pituitary. This accelerates the heartbeat, so the blood circulates more rapidly, and more oxygen flows into the lungs. All these actions speed up the thought processes and supply the body with bursts of energy needed in earlier times for fighting, hunting, and outmaneuvering enemies.

The sympathetic and parasympathetic nerves have another function. Besides regulating the rate of organ function, each acts as a brake on the other if it speeds up too much. The reason these two halves of the autonomic nervous system act in opposite ways is that their acid-alkaline ratios are different. The parasympathetic nerves are predominantly alkaline while the sympathetic nerves are more acidic. When the acid-alkaline balance between these two nerve branches is normal they keep the metabolic functions in balance. But when one half of the autonomic nervous system exerts too much control over the other half, some organs function at too great a speed while others function too slowly. In a few individuals, however, the parasympathetic and sympathetic nerves regulate organ function at about the same rate. These people have balanced metabolisms and so can digest all kinds of protein. Besides the balanced metabolic type, there are two other metabolic types: the parasympathetic dominant, the meat eaters, and the sympathetic dominant, the grain, fish, and fowl eaters.

Kelley's theory on metabolic food typing was built primarily on the research of Emanuel Revici, M.D., and George Watson, Ph.D., both of whom held that the imbalance of certain cellular functions was the cause of disease. Revici believed that in some individuals the regeneration (anabolism) and breakdown (catabolism) of cells don't proceed at the same rate. When this disparity occurs, according to Revici, cellular membranes deteriorate, making it possible for cancer and the AIDS virus to enter cells through tears and holes in cellular membranes. He used injections of fatty acid molecular chains to heal damaged cell membranes. This brought about an equilibrium between the breakdown of cells and their regeneration (catabolic/anabolic function).

Watson, on the other hand, based his metabolic classification on the rate at which cells oxidize (burn food for energy). He believed that in some people the cells burn (oxidize) food too fast while in others, cells burn food too slowly and that either imbalance, if too pronounced, can cause mental disorders. He used diet and nutritional supplements to normalize the rate at which fuel (energy) was used (burned up) in the cells to heal such mental illnesses as chronic depression, bipolar disorder, hyperactivity, and obsessive-compulsive disorders.

Watson's and Revici's theories on the relationship between imbalances in cellular metabolism and disease fit neatly into Kelley's metabolic typing theory based on the imbalance of the autonomic nervous system. To take one example, an individual who is parasympathetic dominant—that is, has excessive digestive stomach acids—is usually also overactive in terms of generating new cells (according to Revici) and burning up fuel (according to Watson). Thus a diet designed to bring about a better balance between the parasympathetic and sympathetic nerve branches also normalizes the speed of oxidation and the regeneration and death (anabolism/catabolism) of cells. In other words, balancing the autonomic nervous system by way of a diet appropriate to the individual's metabolism also takes care of the cellular malfunctions that Revici and Watson contend are the underlying cause of disease.

The Metabolic-Type Diet

Kelley reversed the course of many chronic diseases, including cancer, by lessening the difference between the rate at which the parasympathetic and sympathetic nerves digest food. His choice of diets and nutritional supplements were made on this basis. Since parasympathetic-dominant individuals digest too fast (they have too much stomach acid), Kelley recommended foods such as beef, lamb, pork, and venison because the body breaks them down slowly. This slows the function of organs controlled by the parasympathetic nerves, bringing them closer in line with the rate at which the organs controlled by the sympathetic nerves function.

For the sympathetic-dominant individual, that is, those who digest food too slowly (they have too little stomach acid), Kelley recommends grains as the dietary staple. Grains are broken down fast, forcing the sympathetic nerves to accelerate the body's slow rate of digestion. Those individuals whose parasympathetic and sympathetic nerve branches are balanced can eat all kinds of protein. There is some variation within each of the three metabolic types. When all the organs are functioning at the same rate of speed, the body is said to be in a state of homeostasis.

Another method for individualizing diet is based on blood type. Dr. Peter J. D'Adamo, N.D., postulated that blood type O, the oldest blood type, developed in response to the meat diet of the hunter-gatherer before the cultivation of grains began in various parts of the world between nine thousand and eleven thousand years ago. Type O individuals, like their meat-eating ancestors, according to D'Adamo, need large amounts of meat and small quantities of carbohydrates. In fact, type O individuals, with their high levels of stomach acids needed for breaking down meat, have a tendency toward an underactive thyroid and need vigorous exercise. They fit the profile of Kelley's parasympathetic-dominant metabolic type. (Kelley, however, recommends meat, fat, and butter for the parasympathetic dominant, whereas D'Adamo suggests lean meat for individuals with blood type O.)

Blood type A, according to D'Adamo, represents an adaptation to the cultivation of grains. Blood type A's need for grains and light exercise, and its slow rate of digestion, fit the profile of the sympathetic dominant. Blood type B, D'Adamo states, evolved as a result of the migration of tribes to colder climates. It would also seem to represent an adaptation to dairy products and could explain why so many Asian Indians, with their long history of drinking cow's milk, have blood type B.

The Logic Behind the Meat Eater–Grain Eater Diet Plan

When the individual is in a poor state of health, it's a sign that the systems of the body aren't functioning at normal speed. The first step in normalizing the rate at which the organ systems function is to normalize the speed of digestion. This is where the meat eater–grain eater diet plan comes in. When the individual is eating the foods right for her, the rate of digestion is normalized, so acid waste levels drop and acid-alkaline pHs in the fluids throughout the body become balanced. As a result, *the speed at which the organ systems function returns to normal.*

Before implementing the meat eater–grain eater diet plan, test your acid levels (see the Metabolic-Type Niacin Test that follows). This self-test indicates whether your stomach acid levels are excessive, deficient, or normal. (In the latter case, the individual should eat all kinds of protein so as to keep digestive acid levels stabilized.) If you have an excess of stomach acid, you digest food too fast. In that case, you need the meat eater's diet. Red meat, by taking a long time to digest, slows excessively speedy digestion. At the same time, acid levels stabilize because when too rapid digestion slows down, the excessive acid is used up.

The grain eater's diet addresses the opposite problem—too little stomach acid. Grain, fowl, and fish, by speeding up the grain eater's sluggish digestion, make it possible for the grain eater's deficient acid levels to complete digestion. Once the rate of digestion is normalized,

THE METABOLIC-TYPE NIACIN TEST

To find out whether his patients were grain eaters, meat eaters, or had a balanced metabolism, Kelley had them answer hundreds of questions in a bound book. But he also used a simpler test that he said works equally well. Here it is:

➤ Swallow a 50 mg niacin tablet with water on an empty stomach. The acid-based niacin on top of an excessive acid level in the stomach is bound to cause a reaction. If within a half hour your skin turns red and you feel very hot and itchy, and possibly also experience vaginal itchiness, you know you have a meat-eating metabolism. On the other hand, if the niacin makes you feel warmer, have better color, and feel euphoric, you have a balanced metabolism. If you feel nothing after taking the niacin, you have a grain-eating metabolism.

➤ If you feel the need to confirm the first test, take 8 g of vitamin C a day three days in a row. If you feel depressed, lethargic, exhausted, and irritable, or if you are a woman and experience vaginal irritation, then you have a meat-eating metabolism. If you don't notice any change at all, you have a balanced metabolism. If you feel an improvement—more energy, better quality of sleep—you have a grain-eating metabolism.[6]

all the other internal processes in the body fall in line and proceed at normal speed. When this happens, homeostasis has been achieved and the body has healed itself.

Nutrition for the Meat Eater

If you are parasympathetic dominant and therefore a fast digester, you have large quantities of hydrochloric acid in your stomach, so you should eat red meat frequently. Also limit your intake of such acidic nutrients as vitamin C, lemon juice, and vinegar as well as fruit so as not to speed up your already too rapid digestion of protein. You also have high levels of potassium in relation to calcium. This indicates you should limit the amount of green, leafy vegetables in your diet, since these foods are high in potassium. Generous amounts of calcium will also help bring potassium levels into better balance. Vitamins that should be taken in limited quantities because they speed up the meat eater's already too rapid digestion are B_1, B_2, B_3 in the form of niacin, and B_6; limit the intake of these vitamins to 50 mg each daily.

Nutritional supplements and foods that should be eaten because they slow the meat eater's hyperactive digestion include peas, green beans, cauliflower, and root vegetables with the exception of well-cooked potatoes, which are digested quickly, as well as the nutrients phosphorus, B_3 in the form of niacinamide, inositol, choline, pantothenic acid, and B_{15}.

CAROLINE: THE CLASSIC MEAT EATER

Caroline, age twenty-five, was adopted by a German couple from an orphanage in Seoul, South Korea, and was raised in Finland. She became an accomplished pianist, and by the time she was twenty-one she was giving piano recitals at festivals all over Europe. One of these festivals took place in Salzburg, Austria, where she stayed in the apartment of a friend and cooked her own meals.

One night she broiled a steak she had bought at a butcher shop that purchased its meat supply from an organic farm outside

continued

the city. A few minutes after she finished eating the steak, her lips began to burn and her tongue swelled up so much she said later she felt like someone had stuffed a golf ball in her mouth. A neighbor rushed her to the hospital where she went into anaphylactic shock. Her circulation had slowed so much it caused a sudden drop in her blood pressure, and her pulse could barely be detected. A steroid hormone injection saved her life. The cause of her near death turned out to be the vitamin C preservative in the meat.

Caroline had unusually high acid levels in her stomach even for someone with a meat eater's metabolism. Her already excessive stomach acid levels, increased by the acidity of vitamin C, caused her to go into shock.

Nutrition for the Grain Eater

If you are a grain eater (sympathetic dominant), you are deficient in stomach acid and therefore break down protein too slowly. You should eat generous portions of the foods that the parasympathetic dominant should eat very little of. Besides grains, the sympathetic dominant does well on fowl and fish. Generous amounts of potassium will help lower the high calcium levels of the sympathetic dominant and speed up the burning of fuels. Also take more of those nutrients—niacin, magnesium, folic acid, and vitamin C—that break down fast. Unlike the parasympathetic-dominant meat eater, the sympathetic-dominant grain eater can eat large amounts of green, leafy vegetables; fruit; broccoli; potatoes; and onions. The grain eater's sluggish digestion demands that he or she take slow-digesting nutrients such as choline and B_{15} in small amounts.

Food Allergies

Finding your metabolic type and following up with an appropriate diet doesn't always do away with health problems because it's possible to be allergic to foods even though they're suited to your metabolic type. For example, I'm a meat eater but am allergic to calcium and most of the B vitamins, as well as carrot juice, all food items recommended for the parasympathetic, meat-eating metabolism.

OLEG: THE CLASSIC GRAIN EATER

I was seated next to Oleg at a dinner party put on by the financial services company he worked for. As Oleg gazed at the buffet table, which held immense quantities of rich, overcooked food he had already eaten too much of, he was reminded of the simple foods he had eaten as a youngster growing up in the Ukraine. They never gave him the stomachache that plagued him now.

He began reminiscing about his childhood. Oleg's father, Peter, like his neighbors, raised his own chickens. His family's house was on a street where there were some empty lots. During the day all the chickens in the neighborhood marched en masse to the fields that had grown up inside these lots. There they ate grass and hunted for pieces of calcium-rich limestone. As the sun was beginning to set, the chickens, like homing pigeons, found their way back to the houses of their masters. No identification tags were necessary. For their evening meal, wheat and barley seeds were thrown on the ground, along with loads of sand, which the chickens rooted through for limestone. Oleg remembers that these chickens— every part of which he and his family ate—had a wonderful taste and the eggs the hens laid were a rich orange color like no other egg he has eaten since.

Oleg was aware of the fact that if he was still eating the food he had eaten as a child in the Ukraine he wouldn't have the digestive ailments he was now plagued with, and this was a powerful factor in his decision to go on a metabolically appropriate diet. Another was a family history of diabetes. Every member of his mother's family had become diabetic in their midforties. Oleg was thirty-five. He pictured himself in five or ten years. If he didn't change his eating habits, he knew he would be much fatter by then and would probably also be diabetic. What good would all his money do him then? Oleg took the niacin test and discovered he had a grain-eating metabolism. He went on the grain eater's diet and in two months lost thirty pounds. By the end of a year he had lost an additional twenty pounds and no longer suffered from acid indigestion.

A nearly foolproof method for detecting allergies is the pulse test. Dr. Arthur Coca discovered that food allergies increase the pulse when he noticed that whenever his wife ate certain foods she had an angina attack and her pulse raced.[7] His wife's heart problems disappeared after she eliminated the foods that increased her pulse rate.

In the course of using the pulse test to uncover food allergies, Coca discovered that a whole range of illnesses including migraines, epilepsy, obesity, ulcers, emotional problems, hypertension, asthma, and diabetes could be caused by food allergies because, after eliminating allergy-causing foods, these health problems practically always disappeared.

THE PULSE TEST

This test reveals allergies to particular foods. Before you do any allergy testing, find out the normal range of your pulse rate by taking your pulse for one week before rising (while lying down), just before each meal, and again before going to bed. To take your pulse, place the first two fingers of the right hand on the left wrist. Use a watch or clock with a second hand. Wait until the second hand reaches sixty, and then count the beats until the second hand has returned to sixty (one minute). If you have any problems taking your pulse, use a blood pressure device that also measures pulse rate. If your highest pulse count every day for a week is not over eighty-four and if it is the same each day, you probably don't have any food allergies.

When you are ready to test for allergies, test one food at a time—for example a banana, oatmeal, or a plain slice of bread. Take your pulse just before eating, one-half hour after eating, and one hour after that. Don't eat anything the night before you begin testing for foods. If you are a smoker, don't smoke while you are testing your pulse for allergies.

Coca is vague about the number of beats above the normal rate that indicates an allergy. I have found that if your pulse one-half hour after eating a single food is four to five beats higher than before eating, you're having an allergic reaction to that particular food.

From my experience, blood pressure readings in individuals over fifty are just as accurate a test for allergies as the pulse test and are easier to measure, especially if you take your blood pressure with an electrical device. (Don't use a battery-run blood pressure machine, however, because it gives inaccurate readings when the battery is running down.) A blood pressure reading taken one-half hour after eating that is over 135/85, provided your normal blood pressure is 130/80 or less, is an indication of an allergic reaction to the food you are testing. Any time your blood pressure, after eating a particular food, is four or five degrees higher than it normally is, you know that you are allergic to that food. The higher the blood pressure reading—like the more accelerated the pulse rate—the more allergic you are to it.

One of the most impressive cures through food allergy prevention was that of a multiple sclerosis (MS) patient of Dr. Milo G. Meyer of Michigan City, Indiana.[8] This MS victim, a young man, smoked non-stop all day. He was already badly crippled; he was not able to negotiate the stairs or hold up a baseball bat. After smoking, his pulse rate would zoom upward from sixty-eight to ninety-two beats per minute. This convinced him to give up smoking. Five days after he had done so, he could play baseball with his son and go up and down the stairs without holding the banister. This man's complete recovery from MS—four years later he was still free of the disease—is not an isolated success story. A report by Coca and Meyer describes the elimination of MS in fourteen of fifteen cases by an antiallergy program.

Even if you haven't been diagnosed with a health problem, if you have such "minor" symptoms as fatigue, sleeplessness, mild indigestion, dry eyes, constipation, headaches, or restlessness, you should test yourself for food allergies, particularly those foods that you eat most often, since these are the ones you are most likely to have developed a reaction to.

The Four-Day Rotation Diet

The four-day rotation diet, like the grain eater–meat eater diet plans, improves digestion by optimizing the levels of food-digesting chemicals in the gastrointestinal tract. But while the meat eater–grain eater plan normalizes stomach acid levels—important because acid initiates the breakdown of protein—Theron Randolph's four-day rotation diet (see Randolph's book in the Bibliography) normalizes the protein-digesting enzymes, which complete the digestion of protein.

Randolph's four-day rotation diet works well in terms of increasing food-digesting enzyme levels, because, with no single food eaten more than once every five days, digestive enzymes involved in the breakdown of protein, carbohydrates, and fats have a chance to build up. In the four-day rotation diet even fats and oils are rotated. For example, butter on day one, olive oil on day two, the third day coconut oil, and on the fourth, grapeseed oil. On the fifth day the cycle starts all over again. You go back to butter as well as all the other food items you ate on day one.

Before you start the four-day rotation diet, give up caffeine, alcohol, and cigarettes, and for the first three months avoid those foods you eat three or more times a week, since it's the foods eaten most frequently that are likely to cause allergies. Dr. William Philpott, a neurologist who specialized in magnets, was so enthusiastic about the four-day rotation diet that when people called him to order magnets, before he took their order he urged them to go on this diet. Philpott himself was one of its beneficiaries. According to his wife he was healthier at age eighty-nine than he was at fifty—before he went on the rotation diet that cured him of type 2 diabetes and arthritis.

Randolph's diet is especially effective in reversing type 2 diabetes, which nowadays strikes young adults as well as the middle-aged, prob-ably because by the age of thirty most people are deficient in enzymes. When type 2 diabetics go on Randolph's diet, they increase their enzyme reserves. This helps in the disposal of blood sugar that cannot infiltrate the cells, a problem endemic in type 2 diabetics. Although the beta cells in the pancreas continue to secrete insulin, in type 2 diabetes there is an insulin-resistance problem. I suspect it is not insulin that prevents the cell's absorption of glucose, but the glucose transport car-riers within the cells. In type 2 diabetes, these carriers cannot move from the interior of the cell to the cell membrane to help the glucose molecules pass through the cell's receptors (entry points).

Thus glucose's transportation into the cells depends not only on insulin but also on the transportation system inside the cell. When kept from entering the cells, glucose accumulates in the blood. The four-day rotation diet, by ensuring an adequate supply of enzymes and insulin, prevents the high blood sugar that causes diabetes.

The four-day rotation diet is especially effective in individuals who build up acidic wastes because of digestive juice deficiencies. But it is less effective in cases where degenerative disease is caused by allergic reactions. Multiple sclerosis—the deterioration of the myelin sheathing on the nerve cells—is an example of a disease in which maladaptive reaction to foods is nearly always caused by allergies. That's because it usually strikes individuals in their thirties—at an age when most individuals, while experiencing a drop in digestive enzyme levels, still have enough that they haven't developed serious digestion problems. Thus the first step in the program to reverse the course of MS should be allergy testing. If this doesn't work, try the four-day rotation diet. The key to the success of the four-day rotation diet is the rotation of foods rather than the kind of foods eaten.

The Role of Enzymes

Even before Dr. Kelley devised individual diet plans according to metabolic type, like Max Gerson, he had accomplished a significant number of cancer cures by putting all his patients on the same diet. I knew two of his patients whom he had successfully treated with a standard diet in conjunction with enzymes and juicing: an elderly lady, considered terminally ill with lung cancer, and an airline pilot. Kelley had seemingly cured the pilot of liver cancer. At the end of five years, however, he had a recurrence. Kelley assured him that these were simply residual cancer cells and he'd be fine if he stopped eating meat that had been injected with hormones. It has been several years since he put Kelly's advice into practice, and he hasn't had a recurrence.

The success of the diets of Gerson, Kelley, and Nicholas Gonzales, Kelley's successor, is due to their emphasis on enzymes. They not only prescribed lots of pancreatic enzyme supplements with meals but also made solid and juiced vegetables and fruit (eaten raw to preserve their enzyme content) the cornerstone of their diet regimen. In doing so, they revived a practice based on the discovery of a nineteenth-century Scottish embryologist, Dr. John Beard, who developed the theory that pancreatic enzymes could destroy cancer cells. Dr. Nicholas Gonzalez, M.D., in an interview in the March–April 2000 issue of *New Life* magazine, stated that in the 1920s a number of physicians in the United States and Europe successfully used enzyme treatment for cancer.[9] With the discovery of radiation, however, Beard's enzyme protocol was forgotten.

The emphasis on raw fruit and vegetables worked to the advantage of Kelley's and Gerson's cancer patients for several reasons. First, by supplying the digestive system with enough protein-digesting enzymes to break down the protein in the diet, the protein-digesting enzymes produced by the pancreas were free to kill off cancer cells. Second, since large quantities of low-calorie fruit and vegetables must be eaten to satisfy hunger, they supply the body with large quantities of enzymes. Third, solid fruit and combination fruit and vegetable juice detoxify the liver and neutralize the acidic-waste-filled fluid that cancer cells feed on.

But fruit and vegetables are low in calories, so they have correspondingly low enzyme levels. They are nevertheless the best source of enzymes for cancer patients who can't eat large quantities of raw meat, dairy products, and raw, unfiltered honey, all of which are rich in enzymes.

When my maternal grandfather was an engineering student at the University of Berlin, he developed indigestion. He undertook a cure by eating nothing but raw beef (steak tartare) for several months and had no more stomach problems thereafter. Until the end of his life, my grandfather made what he referred to as scraped meat once a week. He used round steak because of its low fat content, and he scraped the meat from the fiber with his hunting knife. He then added the yolk of a raw egg to the mixture and spread it on buttered brown bread topped with raw onions. The raw beef cured my grandfather's indigestion by supplying his digestive system with the protein-digesting enzymes that the overworked, malfunctioning enzyme-production machinery in his pancreas was not producing in sufficient quantities. The raw beef cure was not my grandfather's idea. At the time he was a young man living in Germany, in the late nineteenth and early twentieth centuries, physicians understood that raw foods had healing properties and used them as therapeutic agents to cure disease.

In 1930, the German government passed legislation to the effect that honey was not to be sold for table use unless it contained the starch-digesting enzyme amylase. The Netherlands passed a similar law in 1925.

In the United States there has never been a law prohibiting the removal of amylase from honey. One might expect brands of honey sold in health-food stores to contain amylase, but most of this honey is clear, an indication that the pollen in which amylase is found has been filtered out.

While honey is the best source of the starch-digesting enzyme amylase, the raw cow's milk cheese sold in many health-food stores is a rich source of the fat-digesting enzyme lipase and protease, a protein-digesting enzyme. The high fat content of cheese, however, makes it wise to follow the folk wisdom of the cheese-loving Dutch: "At breakfast, cheese is gold, at lunch it is silver, and at dinner it is lead." Eating this high-fat dairy product in the morning and at noon, but not in the evening, agrees with the digestive process. In the daytime the body digests and absorbs food quickly, but in the evening and at night digestion slows down.

It was common for physicians in the early part of the twentieth century to use raw milk and butter made from raw milk for therapeutic purposes. Raw milk has a cortisone-like factor that prevents stiffness in the joints.[10] It was also used by physicians to alleviate the symptoms of diabetes until insulin came into use. Louis Pasteur discovered that milk heated to 140 degrees for one-half hour was enough to kill bacteria without destroying any of the nutrients. Port Madison Goat's milk farm in the Seattle area follows this procedure to preserve some of the enzymes in the milk. Their baby goats thrive on goat's milk heated at 140 degrees but get sick if the milk is heated to 160 degrees. Given the deterioration in health of newborn goats who are fed milk just 20 degrees hotter than Pasteur's infection-preventive 140 degrees, how healthy could it be for human babies to be fed milk steam heated at the boiling temperature of 212 degrees? This is the temperature at which the agribusiness dairies heat their milk.

At this temperature practically all the nutrients in the milk are destroyed as is the acidity needed to break down the calcium.[11] The purpose of boiling the milk at 212 degrees is not to keep the public safe from disease-causing bacteria but to extend the shelf life of the product. The law, which requires pasteurization of milk to kill off bacteria, should prohibit the heating of milk for purposes that have nothing to do with the prevention of infectious disease. A brand of milk that seems to last forever in the refrigerator has been heated at such a high temperature that all its nutrients have been destroyed. Five years ago I noticed that during the summer, even some nonorganic milk in my refrigerator spoiled. Now even the organic milk I buy doesn't spoil in the summer (with the exception of a brand of milk called Eco Meal). It would seem that almost all brands of milk are boiled at such a high temperature that no nutrients are left to spoil.

Fats and Oils

Most doctors recommend that only 10 to 15 percent of the diet consist of fat because they believe it to be a major factor in colon and rectal cancer, the second leading causes of cancer-related deaths in the United States. It was therefore a shock to the medical community when two studies involving thousands of individuals indicated that a low-fat, high-fiber diet did not reduce the incidence of colon cancer.[12]

These studies assumed that a low-fat diet, like a high-fiber one, is a colon and rectal cancer preventative—based on the assumption that a high-fat diet is conducive to the development of cancer. A study found that women on a low-fat diet had the same rate of breast cancer as women who consumed large quantities of fat.[13] What isn't considered is the fact that soluble fibers cannot neutralize carcinogens unless they are first absorbed by fat in the colon. It seems likely, therefore, that the low-fat, high-fiber diet didn't reduce colon cancer because there was not enough fat to absorb the carcinogenic substances in the intestines.

High-fat diets have also been linked to cardiovascular disease because it is assumed that the fat the body doesn't use sticks to the walls of arteries and hardens. In fact, fatty cholesterol adheres to arterial walls because these walls have already sustained injuries. The layering of fat over inflamed, scratched, and bruised arterial walls is simply a response mechanism, designed to protect the arteries from developing leaks and hemorrhaging.

One of the more likely causes of artery deterioration was revealed in a study done in 1972 at the University of Hawaii with pigs as subjects. Eighty-five percent of the pigs fed high levels of sugar developed heart disease, while the pigs fed a diet in which 10 percent of the sugar was replaced by coconut oil or beef tallow retained normal heart function. It seems that the small percentage of fat fed to the pigs actually protected their arteries from the sharp, acidic crystals of sugar.

Fat, along with carbohydrates and protein, is one of the basic food types that the body requires to sustain itself. The body itself has a high fat content. Aside from water, there is more fat in the body than any other substance. Cellular membranes that cover the cell are made up almost entirely of fatty acid (the form of fat into which the fat we eat is broken down), and the brain is more than 60 percent fatty acid. Moreover, fatty acids, along with protein (in the form of amino acids) play a vital role in the manufacture of energy. Transportation of oxygen by the red blood cells would not be possible without the fatty acid–protein membrane covering the red blood cell through which oxygen gains entry into the cell.

There is evidence that too little fat is harmful to the body. When Max Gerson began using nutrition to treat cancer, the diet he recommended contained only fats and oils that were intrinsic to the food. Later on he included fat and oil supplements and got a better rate of recovery. Mental as well as physical health is dependent on the consumption of enough fats and oils. This is shown in studies in which children with emotional disorders who were put on a low-fat diet became more aggressive and violent.[14]

Given the role of fat in the production of cellular energy, hormones, and bile; in blood clotting; in the digestion of meat protein; and in immune system function, a more realistic ratio of fat in relation to the other food types in the diet is 25 to 30 percent. A study at MIT using human subjects concluded that the ratio of the three main food types should be the following: carbohydrates 60 percent, fat 25 percent, and protein 15 percent. Establishing the minimum daily fat requirement leads to the next problem, namely, the kinds of fat the body needs. Cellular membranes contain saturated, monounsaturated, and polyunsaturated fats, while the brain structure is made up of a mix of saturated and polyunsaturated fats of the omega-3 family, such as docosahexaenoic acid (DHA), and the omega-6 family, such as arachidonic acid (AA).

The wide range of fatty acids in the body point out the variety of fats and oils we should eat to satisfy the body's fat requirements. The fatty acid requirements of the brain are one part omega-3 oils (found in saltwater fish; green, leafy vegetables; and eggs) to four parts omega-6 fats (found in meat and polyunsaturated oils). (Don't satisfy your omega-6 fatty acid requirements by including corn, soy, and safflower oils in your diet. These oils should be avoided, since they raise stress hormone levels and are associated with cancer.)

Fats and Oils for the Meat Eater

Should deficiencies in omega-3 oils be overcome by consuming large quantities of green, leafy vegetables and saltwater fish and limiting the consumption of meat and omega-6 polyunsaturated oils? It depends on your metabolic type. If you have a meat-eating metabolism, eating meat four or five times a week, which includes a moderate amount of meat fat, is healthy—provided the meat contains no hormones or pesticides. As a meat eater, you are limited in the amount of green, leafy vegetables (omega-3 fatty acid) you can eat. But eating green, leafy vegetables once a week, salad three times weekly, and saltwater fish once a week should satisfy the meat eater's omega-3 fatty acid requirements. Avoid corn, safflower, and cottonseed oils so as not to raise omega-6 fatty acid levels in your brain, which has the effect of raising stress hormone levels. Meat eaters do well on large quantities of butter and can also use olive oil on their salad.

Fats and Oils for the Grain Eater

It's easier for the grain-eating metabolic type to balance omega-6 and omega-3 fatty acids, since grain eaters do well on large amounts of green, leafy vegetables. Fish is also compatible with the grain eater's metabolism. Like the meat eater, the grain eater should avoid corn, safflower, and cottonseed oils not only because of the omega-6 overload in the brain but also because they give off toxic lipid peroxides. Studies show an increase in the rate of cancer among heavy users of omega-6 polyunsaturated vegetable oils. Long-chain oils were less of a problem before grains were refined because the vitamin E in whole grains helped neutralize the toxins generated by polyunsaturated oils as they are broken down into fatty acids.

Margarine and mayonnaise, made from oils that have been hydrogenated, should be avoided. During the process of hydrogenation all the nutrients are removed from the oil, so the digestive system must rob the body's store of nutrients to break down the empty calories in the hydrogenated oil. Hydrogenation also leaves behind trace amounts of aluminum and nickel, which may find their way into the brain and contribute to the development of Alzheimer's disease.

Rancid oil is another problem. French fries and doughnuts in fast-food restaurants are deep fried in oil that has been used over and over again and in the process has become rancid, and therefore carcinogenic. Moreover, the temperature of the oil in which these foods are cooked is so high the structure of the fat molecules in the food is altered. Misshapen molecules become rigid and elongated. After being absorbed into the cells, they stiffen the cells' membranes. Some scientists believe this could give rise to emotional problems and learning disabilities in children because rigid cell membranes could interfere with the transmission of thoughts between brain cells.

Any food whose molecular structure is altered is carcinogenic. But as far as other fats and oils are concerned, it's not so easy to label them either good or bad. For example, if you take vitamin E supplements when you eat polyunsaturated vegetable oils, they lose most of their toxicity. On the other hand, long-term use of vitamin E, shorn of its cofactors, removes calcium from the bones. An example of a very healthy oil that under certain conditions can become toxic is the oil in fish. To make fish oil available to the body and to prevent it from becoming toxic, short-chain fats like butter or medium-chain oils like coconut oil should be eaten along with the fish. These shorter-chain fats and oils act like scissors, cutting up the long molecular chains in fish oil into pieces that are small enough to be absorbed through cell membranes. Butter is also beneficial because it contains short chains of butyric fatty acid that are burned up rather than stored as fat.

Coconut oil is easily burned up, thus providing the body with an efficient form of fuel that is also good for weight loss. In addition, coconut oil keeps the energy-producing factories in the cells—the mitochondria—in good repair. Furthermore, coconut oil can be heated to a very high temperature without having its atomic structure altered. According to the chemist Ray Peat, Ph.D., coconut oil is a very effective cancer preventive. People have a hard time believing that it has so many health benefits given that it is supersaturated. But a saturated fat with single bonds that bind atoms together doesn't break down and become toxic when it is subjected to heat the way the double- and triple-bonded (polyunsaturated) oils do.

Meat fat is also stable because it contains saturated and monounsaturated fatty acids. I knew a healthy woman in her late nineties who ate fatty meat and cream sauce made with butter every day. She claimed the meat was more easily digested if eaten with butter. Her intuition was correct because the short-chain fatty acids in butter break apart the long-chain saturated fats in meat, making them available to the body for energy production.

It's advisable, however, to avoid eating large quantities of meat fat because the enzyme lipase used to break down the meat fat is destroyed when meat is cooked. Authors of books on holistic nutrition wax enthusiastic about the cardiovascular health of the traditional Eskimos who ate whale and seal fat as if it were candy. But the Eskimos ate their fat raw. Raw fat leaves behind practically no acetone, the toxic by-product of cooked fat that can cause degeneration of the heart and arteries.

In the winter my husband and I often eat roast duck at a Hungarian restaurant on the upper east side of Manhattan. We felt we were damaging our arteries, eating what was essentially nine-tenths saturated fat and one-tenth meat—until I read that in the Gascony region of France where people are known for their longevity, duck and goose fat make up almost all the fat in the diet. People in this region cook everything in duck fat, snack on fried duck skin, spread goose or duck fat on bread, and eat liver pâté (foie gras), which is 87 percent duck or goose fat. Despite this high intake of cooked, saturated fat that contains no fat-digesting lipase, out of 100,000 middle aged Frenchmen in this region, only 80 die of heart attacks yearly, whereas in the rest of France the number is 145. In the United States, 315 out of 100,000 middle-aged men die of heart attacks each year.[15] Further proof that the longevity of people in this region—ninety-five-year-olds are common—is due to their consumption of duck and goose fat is the fact that in a part of the region where people eat the most fat, having foie gras three or four times weekly, they live longer than in areas where foie gras is eaten only once a week. Scientists speculate that the health benefits of duck and goose fat could be due to the similarity of their molecular structure to that of olive oil.

The low death rates from heart disease of people who eat duck and goose fat, however, could also be due to their custom of drinking one or two glasses of red or white wine, an equal amount of mineral water, and a salad whenever they eat duck or goose.

Olive oil has received a great deal of favorable publicity in recent years. Some people refer to it as the miracle oil because of the longevity of the inhabitants of the islands off the coasts of Italy, Greece, and Spain who consume huge amounts of it. In Sardinia, where cancer and heart disease are rare, the inhabitants there drink olive oil by the glassful.

It's doubtful that we could obtain the same healthy arteries by consuming as much olive oil as the people living on these islands do. The oil they drink is greenish, opaque, and thick—whereas the olive oil

---

SOME HEALTHY FATS AND OILS

➤ **Coconut oil.** This supersaturated oil does not increase cholesterol levels because the blood carries it directly to the cells where it is used as fuel to make energy. (All other fats and oils entering the bloodstream are dropped off in the liver, where they are "loaded" onto LDL or HDL carriers and returned to general circulation.) Coconut oil is an excellent cooking oil because it can be heated to a very high temperature without being denatured and becoming carcinogenic. Organic coconut oil is sold in health-food stores.

➤ **Ghee (the liquid part of butter).** This is good for cooking because it doesn't break down. It is used in Ayurvedic medicine, the ancient Indian form of healing, because it is thought to be good for the *ojas* (soul).

➤ **Goose and duck fat.** This fat is healthy for the cardiovascular system. Save the fat given off by the roasting duck or goose. Refrigerate and use as a spread on bread.

➤ **Extra-virgin olive oil.** Two Spanish brands, Columela Picual and Nuñez de Prado, being greenish and opaque, contain more nutrients than clear, yellow olive oil. Unfiltered olive oil prevents artery damage and cancer. You can order these brands through the Whole Foods Market website (wholefoodsmarket.com).

➤ **Freeze-dried vegetables.** The green powder in a jar sold in health-food stores is a great source of omega-3 fatty acid because it's made up mostly of green, leafy vegetables. Two or three spoonfuls in apple juice daily is a good substitute for anyone who doesn't like green, leafy vegetables.

➤ **Butter.** Cultured, unsalted butter is available in most supermarkets as well as in health-food stores.

available in this country, although labeled unfiltered, is yellow and clear, an indication that a great many nutrients have been filtered out of it.

The Role of Fiber

Fiber-rich foods help prevent many degenerative diseases. In the intestines, fibers bind with bile acids so they can't damage the lining of the intestinal walls, and when fiber is broken down, its short-chain fatty acids neutralize carcinogenic substances in the colon. Fibers also help control type 2 diabetes and heart disease. According to a study published in May 2000 in *The New England Journal of Medicine*, type 2 diabetics on a diet with twice the fiber consumed by those in another group of diabetics had more nearly normal levels of blood sugar and insulin as well as lower cholesterol and triglyceride levels.[16]

The individual's choice of fiber must conform to metabolic type. The grain eater is fortunate because grain provides fiber in far more bulk than the raw vegetables from which the meat-eating metabolic types must obtain most of their fiber needs.

HOW FIBER CURED ANGELA'S DIGESTIVE PROBLEMS

Angela, in her early twenties, had suffered painful muscle spasms in her stomach for a year. At the recommendation of a nutritionist she took pancreatic enzymes, and when these didn't help she went to an herbalist. The herbalist prescribed a formula made up of fennel seed, chamomile flowers, dandelion, gentian, and gingerroots. The herbal digestive aid didn't work either.

Had these alternative health-care specialists questioned Angela about her eating habits and considered her ethnic background, they might have discovered the cause of her stomach problems. Before Angela moved to the Seattle area she lived in the desert country west of Tucson with other members of her tribal group, the Seri Indians. When she left the desert, she took with her the craving for hot sauce that Indians living in hot climates have developed. However, lacking the special hot peppers needed to make this hot sauce, Angela ate chili dogs and tortilla chips with salsa. She also ate white rice and white bread in place of the fiber-rich cholla cactus buds, tepary beans, and mesquite that she and the other Indians living in the desert had eaten.

Her new diet lacked the soluble fibers of her traditional diet, which had speeded the transit of hot sauce through her digestive tract, not giving it a chance to irritate her stomach tissues. As it was, her fiber-deficient diet slowed her digestion, leaving behind spicy, acidic food residues that inflamed her stomach muscles and caused them to go into spasms.

Angela began eating oatmeal, seven-grain bread, and sprouted wheat bread for its enzyme content. The fibers, along with the enzyme supplements she was taking, broke down her foods at a faster pace, and the hot, spicy foods moved more quickly through her digestive tract. This gave her inflamed stomach tissues a chance to heal. Soon after, her stomach spasms went away.

Devices to Detoxify the Body

Long before the advent of modern medicine, cultures developed ways to detoxify the body, some of which are still in use today. Indians in the western hemisphere used sweat lodges; one reservation in North Dakota has begun using them again. The Japanese still use hot baths, as do the Greeks, who in ancient times purged themselves seasonally with colonics and regurgitation. While the Scandinavians developed saunas similar to the Indian sweat lodges, the central Europeans used highly mineralized waters and clay wraps to draw the toxins out of the body. Spas are still popular. Until a few years ago, in Germany everyone past sixty-five got two six-week vacations at a spa paid for by the government.

Magnetic and Far Infrared Mattress Pads

Modern technology has made possible the invention of devices for ridding the body of toxins that are far more convenient than many traditional detoxifying practices because they can be used in the course of the day while sleeping or working. One such device is the far infrared mattress pad invented by Japanese scientists. The safe direct current (DC) in the pad (converted from the universal AC) flows through carbon-impregnated sheets, radiating heat waves that penetrate the innermost recesses of the body and dissolve and remove acid wastes—like the sun's red light waves, which ripen fruits and vegetables by lifting out the acid. Of all the heat waves that radiate from the sun, infrared is the safest and most healthy.

While far infrared energy rids the body of waste through its deep, penetrating heat, negatively charged magnetic mattress pads do so through polar force. When you sleep on a magnetic pad or place a magnet anywhere on your body, the positively charged ions in the iron in the hemoglobin in your blood are attracted to the negatively charged ions emitted by the iron in the magnet. When magnets are placed near an injury, this increases the blood supply to the injured area, and this increased blood flow oxygenates the injured tissues, reducing redness and swelling. Dr. Philpott has normalized high blood pressure by using magnetic sleeping pads, which he says work by removing the fatty plaque buildup on artery walls.

Alkaline Water

Alkaline water also rids the body of acidic waste. A water ionizer can separate out the positively charged acidic particles from the negatively charged alkaline particles, resulting in alkaline water for drinking and cooking, and acidic water for washing, since the skin is acidic.[17] You can also buy small bottles of an alkaline solution and add a few drops to foods and liquids. One of my readers was not able to digest any food but brown rice—and even brown rice gave her some digestive problems. She found, however, that she could digest the brown rice well once she sprinkled a few drops of this alkaline solution over it.

Ionizing Air Cleaner

My air cleaner operates on the basis of negative and positive charges (see Resources). Just as negatively and positively charged particles occur in the earth and in water, they are also found in the air. In the purest atmosphere—in the mountains and forests and along the seashore—there are four negatively charged particles for every three positively charged ones. The ionizing air cleaner that I own generates negatively and positively charged ions in the same ratio of four to three as the earth's atmosphere, but it is the negatively charged particles that clean the air. They stick to the positively charged dust particles and other contaminants, and the combined weight causes them to drop to the floor. There is some controversy regarding ozone, but the fact is that the ozone (O_3) generated by this air cleaner oxidizes (burns up) molds, mildew, and airborne bacteria such as the tuberculosis bacillus.

Pure air is invigorating because with the acidic, toxic pollutants removed, it carries more oxygen. This additional oxygen is transported by the blood to the cells, where it is converted by the process of respiration into energy. Increasing the body's energy level not only promotes a sense of well-being but also enables the metabolic processes in the body to work efficiently in eliminating the acidic wastes that lay the groundwork for degenerative diseases.

Vitamin Supplements Can Deplete Nutritional Reserves

There are many misconceptions about vitamin supplements. It's important to know how supplements have the ability to deplete nutritional reserves; keeping this in mind is key when neutralizing your body's acidity.

Some health enthusiasts may talk nostalgically about the wild game, roots, and berries that their remote ancestors, the hunter-gatherers of the Paleolithic Age, lived on. And most assume that the nutritional supplements they take make up the difference between the natural diet of these ancient, Ice Age peoples and the nutrient-deficient, chemicalized foods that make up their own diet. Their belief takes for granted that a single vitamin, mineral, or enzyme is a nutrient and therefore can help restore the body's deficient nutrient reserves.

In fact once a vitamin is separated from the food complex in which it occurs naturally in the body, it loses its nutritional value. Epidemiological studies support this. They show that while the ingestion of fruits and vegetables reduces the risk of cancer, diabetes, and heart disease, such antioxidents as beta-carotene, ascorbic acid, and alpha tocopherol (vitamin E) don't have such health benefits. We need whole-food vitamins. In the case of vitamin E, that includes tocopherols E2, E3, unsaturated fatty acids, F1, F2, xanthene, liposoitols, selenium, coenzyme Q-10, and other factors not yet discovered.[18]

Judith A. DeCava, M.S., LNC, points out in her book *The Real Truth About Vitamins and Antioxidants* the huge number of studies that show the damage to health of single vitamins and minerals. The long-term use of vitamin E without its co-nutrients demineralizes bone calcium, and large amounts of bioflavonoids taken over a long period create a deficiency of the clotting factor vitamin K. Furthermore, longtime use of high-potency vitamin D has been shown to encourage the clogging of the arteries and heart disease. DeCava describes an experiment conducted by F. G. Hopkins, a biochemist, in the early part of the twentieth century. He fed laboratory animals a diet of nothing but refined protein, fat, carbohydrates, minerals, and water. The animals died, while the control group that was fed unprocessed foods thrived. [19]

There is another danger to taking single vitamins. Robbed of their co-nutrients, they have to steal from the body's nutritional reserves. Without this "theft," they would have no curative value. When because of an overconsumption of single vitamins or minerals these reserves are depleted, the condition the vitamin was meant to alleviate may worsen. Fortunately, there are now a number of brands of whole-food nutritional supplements that are sold in health-food stores.

Having pointed out the dangers of taking single vitamins and minerals, I have to call attention to their initial health advantages. They can alleviate many degenerative diseases—but for the sake of your long-term health, observe the following precautions. Along with the single nutrients you take, add a multivitamin whole-food supplement. And once your health problem has cleared up—unless you have major depression or schizophrenia—gradually cut down on your dosage of single nutrients and replace them with whole-food vitamin complexes.

After carefully evaluating the results of my advice to hundreds of individuals, I'm convinced that toxicity in the form of acidic waste is the primary cause of degenerative disease. Unfortunately the health obsession over nutritional supplements obscures the vital role played by the removal of acidic toxins in normalizing organ function. Nutritional supplements are usually necessary to heal injured organs, but it is difficult to heal an organ system until the acidic wastes that caused the injury to the body are first removed.

A diet tailored to the individual's metabolism helps reduce acidic waste levels in the body. With the information contained in this chapter you should be able to find the diet that is right for you. Food items as well as single vitamins and whole-food vitamin complexes for particular health problems are discussed in Part II.

ACHIEVING PH BALANCE TO TREAT SPECIFIC AILMENTS

CHAPTER 3

DIGESTIVE AILMENTS

A cid waste, under ideal conditions, is nothing more than the by-
product of all the physical and chemical processes that go on in
the body. Such acid waste is easily neutralized and removed by way of
sweat, urine, and stool. But when there is—in addition to this naturally
occurring acid waste in the body—acidic waste from the breakdown of
undigested food, the body can't dispose of all of it. In this situation, acid
waste causes health problems. The first to show up is usually acid indigestion, most particularly, acid reflux.

Acid Reflux

Acid reflux, characterized by a burning in the throat and chest, occurs
when the acidic waste from undigested food flows from the stomach
into the esophagus (throat). Unlike the stomach, the esophagus doesn't
have a thick mucous lining to protect it from the harsh acid crystals of
the debris. If acid reflux is chronic, it causes swelling and redness in the
esophageal tissues. This can lead to the erosion of the esophagus and
eventually to cancer. High levels of acid waste in the stomach can trigger such gastric problems as a spastic stomach, duodenal ulcers, and
intestinal inflammation. (The duodenum, the uppermost part of the
small intestine, is attached at the bottom of the stomach.)

Symptoms of acid indigestion can be a lifesaver because they provide
evidence that acidic waste in the digestive tract is reaching dangerous
levels and therefore accumulating in other parts of the body as well.

Sooner or later excessive acid waste gives rise to degenerative disease. Many individuals, however, develop debilitating illness without having any symptoms of acid indigestion; with no gastric symptoms, they don't see the link between poor digestion and diseases in the organ systems outside the digestive tract.

Even those with acid reflux, gastritis (inflammation of the stomach), nausea, bloating, gallstones, and ulcers, where diet is an obvious culprit, find it hard to believe that foods that cause digestive problems can also injure organs not part of the digestive system. Yet every ache and pain in the body that isn't the result of physical injury or genetic predisposition is triggered by the acidic waste products of inappropriate and/or nutrient-deficient food.

Unhappily for their patients, mainstream doctors view symptoms of illness as signs of disease rather than as reactions to metabolically inappropriate foods. Mary was a victim of this approach. Six years ago on her way home from a party, her heart started racing, her hands trembled, and minutes later she had a seizure. Because tests came out negative, the doctor concluded that she had the flu. But instead of getting over the "flu," she developed shivering fits, felt tremendous pressure in her head, and could hardly hold herself up. After she had seven seizures in one week, the doctor conducted more extensive tests. An EEG (electroencephalogram), performed while she slept, showed that her brain waves were off the charts: 1:2 is normal; hers had slowed to 1:600. A blood workup revealed that she had an adrenal insufficiency and her antibodies were so elevated that they were a strong indication of an autoimmune disorder. The doctor suspected lupus. Mary was already taking antiseizure medication and was now told that she should take prednisone, a steroid hormone, and undergo cytotoxin chemotherapy. She decided that these drugs were the proverbial straws that would break the camel's back, in this case hers, so she took matters into her own hands and went to a naturopathic physician. The first thing that the naturopath did was to test for allergies. The tests indicated that Mary was allergic to wheat, sugar, dairy, caffeine, alcohol, bananas, and potatoes. She went on an allergy-free diet, and in a few days her symptoms disappeared. She regained her sense of well-being, alertness, and ability to concentrate two to three weeks later. The nightmare was over. Thinking back on her illness, what frightens her most is the fact that as sick as she was, she had no symptoms of indigestion from her food allergies and therefore no clue as to why she was so ill. Mary's experience shows that the role of diet in initiating an illness should be the first consideration even when there are no symptoms of indigestion.

I would probably have missed this connection myself if years ago when I began having symptoms of acid indigestion I hadn't been teaching the basic 101 course in chemistry for the first time. The timing was fortuitous. Along with my students, I learned that a balance of acidic particles (positively charged protons) and alkaline particles (negatively charged electrons) make up the basic structure of the elements—principally, carbon, nitrogen, oxygen, and hydrogen—out of which all the tissues in the body are made. (Neutrons in the nucleus of atoms have no charge.) When a compound contains more electrons than protons, it is negatively charged (hydroxyl ions, OH-), and when it contains more protons than electrons, it is positively charged (hydrogen ions, H+). This made me realize the full implications of having acid indigestion. If it caused an imbalance in the acid-alkaline ratios of the blood and other fluids in the body, any or all of my organ systems could malfunction and deteriorate.

The Real Cause of Acid Reflux

Doctors have tried to cure acid reflux through surgery, repairing the valve between the stomach and esophagus to keep it from opening up and letting stomach acids pour into the esophagus. In view of the fact that the results of this operation have been disappointing, there has to be another explanation for acid reflux. The most likely one is that acidic waste gas molecules in the stomach open the valve that closes off the stomach from the esophagus by causing it to go into a spasm. (This valve should remain closed except when we eat.) Acidic waste flows through this opening, inflaming the esophagus. Chronic inflammation wears away the esophageal tissues.

Efficient digestion depends on the alternating actions of acid and alkaline digestive juices. The alkaline enzyme ptyalin in the mouth breaks down starch; hydrochloric acid and acidic gastric juices, such as pepsin, break up protein in the stomach; in the small intestine alkaline pancreatic enzymes complete the digestion of protein, and alkaline bile emulsifies fats and oils. Acid reflux can disrupt this acid-alkaline sequence by changing the pH factor in the stomach and small intestine.

How this happens is revealed by the typical contents of the stomach that heartburn sufferers sometimes throw up in an effort to get rid of the burning sensation in the throat and chest. After a highly acidic liquid is brought up, alkaline-forming bile often follows, indicating that the bile has flowed from the small intestine into the stomach, where it doesn't belong. This occurs when the pyloric valve between the stomach and small intestine opens, most likely because the acid waste causes the muscles in the valve to relax. The alkaline-forming bile in the stomach alkalinizes the acidic gastric juices, thus interfering with the stomach's breakdown of protein. As a result not only does the undigested protein turn into acid waste, but the alternating acid-alkaline balance in the digestive tract is disrupted.

The Healing Value of Raw Potatoes

Once I understood how foods that the digestive system can't handle disrupt the acid-alkaline balance in the digestive tract, I figured out what foods gave me acid reflux and eliminated them. These troublesome foods were largely acidic in taste (because of their overabundance of protons): fruit, vinegar, and caffeine, which leaves a sour taste in the mouth. I did well on such alkaline foods as white potatoes, string beans, cauliflower, peas, and other root vegetables. On the other hand, there were alkaline foods such as radishes, mustard, onions, garlic, herbs, and spices I avoided because their bitter, sharp taste irritated my digestive tract.

Thus bland-tasting foods became the staple of my breakfast and lunch; I cook them in a frying pan along with some vegetables in a little water. I drink the water the potatoes and vegetables are cooked in. At first, I ate potatoes and vegetables because they were the only foods I could digest. I never anticipated the miraculous healing effect they would have.

I began by cooking the potatoes until they were soft. Then some instinct told me to cook them less. As I began to feel better I realized it was because I was barely cooking the potatoes, so I cooked them less and less. After I had been on this nearly raw potato diet for a year, I went to a dinner party where the hostess served a highly spiced Spanish concoction of some sort. For the first time in years after eating something so spicy it burned my tongue, I didn't get acid indigestion. A few weeks later I had a pizza with garlic, which also had no effect. My digestive problems gradually became a thing of the past. The occasional stomach upset I have now goes away when I eat a few slices of raw potato. The raw potato also acts as an appetite suppressant, absorbing the acidic wastes in the stomach that can incite hunger.

The alkaline starch in the potatoes had healed my indigestion in part by absorbing and neutralizing the acid waste—which had probably lain in my digestive tract for years. I discovered another component in potatoes involved in this healing when I read a paper that Francis M. Pottenger Jr., M.D., presented at the Thirty-Eighth Annual Meeting of the American Therapeutic Society, in Atlantic City, June 4, 1937.[1] In it he discussed the importance of the gluelike mucilage in raw foods in helping the enzymes in the stomach break down the food mass. This brought to mind that when I ran my fingers along the inside surface of the pan in which I had cooked potatoes, I felt a sticky coating. This was mucilage! The heat from cooking had separated it out from the fiber in the potato. While mucilage is a property of all foods, it is most abundant in okra and raw meat and, as I discovered, is also plentiful in potatoes—provided they are only partially cooked.

The nearly raw potatoes I'd been eating supplied two substances that improved my digestion: water, which enables the food mass in the stomach to absorb the digestive enzyme juices, and mucilage, which by coating the food mass prevents the water from seeping out. Given the vital role played by water and mucilage in the ability of the food mass in the stomach to absorb enzymes, how could a diet of totally cooked food, which has no water and enzymes to speak of, be digested? It can't. Unlike a food mass containing some raw foods, which forms the proper gluelike lump in the stomach, a mass of cooked food forms distinct layers: cooked meat, the heaviest, on the bottom; bread or cake next; then a layer of vegetables, and mashed potatoes interspersed through the three layers.

Rapid digestion that leaves a minimum of food debris can't take place unless enzymes are able to penetrate the food mass, and this isn't possible unless some raw foods, with their supply of water and mucilage, are eaten at every meal. Mucilage also heals the stomach lining and builds up the layer of mucus that covers it. I'm convinced it was the thickening of this mucous layer from the mucilage in potatoes that has made my stomach impervious to the irritating effects of spicy foods. It makes sense that potatoes—with their high level of mucilage—can help in the regrowth of the mucus that had lined the stomach before bad diet destroyed it. Potatoes were used by tribal cultures to heal skin irritations and wounds. The American Indians placed a slice of raw potato on the eyelid to heal pinkeye, and in West Africa herbalists covered the incisions they made— for example, when they cut a circular-shaped piece out of the skull in order to drain fluid from the brain—with raw potato slices.

The nearly raw potato diet can take anywhere from two months to a year and a half to work. The less you cook the potatoes the faster the healing process. You can speed up healing by drinking a glass of raw potato juice every day or eating slices of peeled, raw potatoes. Although potatoes are digested quickly, even those who digest their foods too fast (the parasympathetic-dominant meat eater) can do well on the semiraw potato diet, because potatoes that are barely cooked are broken down slowly. Raw potatoes not only improve digestion by reducing acidity but also heal stomach injuries—ulcers, lesions, and inflammation (gastritis)—by building up the protective mucous lining of the stomach.

Although regarded by nutritionists as unhealthy because of their high levels of starch, the more than 150 studies on the white potato present a more sanguine view of this root vegetable. Perhaps most significant is the fact that the starch in potatoes differs from the starch in grains in that it is broken down not by digestion but rather by fermentation in the large intestine. As a result, blood sugar remains low, an indication that potatoes act as a preventative of diabetes and cardiovascular disease. Further benefits occur as white potatoes ferment. They give off two substances, one that decreases the appetite and the other, an acid, that lines the colon with an anticancer substance.[2]

Potatoes are not only good medicine but also have enormous nutritional value. This was proven when this protein-rich carbohydrate almost single-handedly kept the Irish alive for a 150-year period. Potatoes became the dietary staple of the Irish with the final takeover of Northern Ireland by the British in 1690 in the battle of the Boyne. The most fertile land was given to the officers of the victorious British army, and Irish farmers were forced to plant potatoes, the only crop that would grow on the barren soil left to them. The potato blight of 1843 put an end to the consumption of potatoes for many years by destroying every potato crop in Ireland.

What few people are aware of is that potatoes kept the Germans from starving after World War I when their economy lay in ruins. Another little-known fact about potatoes is that on board ships in the nineteenth century, they were more effective in healing and preventing scurvy than limes. A small village in Japan, where the dietary staple is white potatoes, currently has the longest documented life span in the world. (More information on this village is found in my book *Eat Right for Your Metabolism*.)

Gelatin Supplies Mucilage

Pottenger mentioned powdered okra and beet juice as effective hydrophilic colloids (sticky substances that have an affinity for water) but believed the most practical and effective musilagenous substance was gelatin taken with each meal, either sprinkled on food or added to liquid. For an individual with alcoholic-related gastritis, gelatin with its enormous mucilage content is often the only remedy that will counteract the corrosive effect of alcohol on the lining of the stomach and small intestine. Gelatin also has great nutritive value, an additional benefit for alcoholics who have lost interest in food. Edgar Cayce in one of his readings stated that gelatin aids in the absorption of vitamins and minerals. Dr. Bernard Jensen in *Foods That Heal* writes that because the calcium in gelatin (45 percent of gelatin consists of calcium) is derived from chicken bones, it's the most easily assimilated form of that mineral.[3]

Ulcers

My mother was fed cow's milk as a baby and continued to drink it until, at the age of five, the chronic rash on her face and arms was diagnosed as an allergic reaction to milk. I suspect that the gallbladder attacks she began having in her early thirties were caused by the same chemical and/or immune system imbalance that had caused her allergy to milk as a child.

She relieved her painful gallbladder attacks, brought on by gall-stones, with a hot water bottle, and the nausea that accompanied these attacks with an alkaline concoction made up of peppermint, spirits of ammonia, and sodium bicarbonate in water. A surgeon, a friend of the family, talked her into having her gallbladder removed by assuring her that, because the gallbladder's only function was storing bile, it was expendable. (In fact, when the gallbladder is removed, the liver inter-prets this act as a sign that bile is no longer needed to digest fats, so it curtails its production of bile.) After removing the gallbladder, the surgeon did some exploratory surgery and discovered, much to his horror, that every inch of the lining of her stomach and duodenum (the upper part of the small intestine) was covered with ulcers. He told my mother after the operation that he regretted having taken out her gallbladder—despite the pain her gallbladder, left intact, would con-tinue to give her—because the diet for ulcers (at the time) emphasized milk, butter, and cream. These dairy products can be digested only with the help of the large quantity of bile that can be stored in the gallbladder, so without her gallbladder my mother wouldn't have enough bile to break down the fat in butter and cream. And without this fat her ulcers wouldn't heal—or so the medical profession thought at the time. The result was that her gallbladder attacks worsened and her ulcers became seemingly permanent fixtures in her stomach and duodenum.

The Healing Quality of Raw Cabbage Juice

When my mother was in her late eighties, she finally agreed to try a natural cure for her ulcers and gallbladder attacks—raw cabbage juice. Reluctantly, she began drinking two pints of it a day, sometimes adding carrots. In only two weeks she began having fewer stomach upsets. Two months later she stopped having them altogether.

The effectiveness of raw cabbage in healing ulcers—as well as elimi-nating gallstones—proves that foods that contain more acid-forming minerals than alkaline ones, despite the claims otherwise, can heal the body. Raw cabbage cleans out the acid waste in the stomach, allowing ulcers to heal and the mucous membrane lining in the stomach to rebuild itself. The beneficial action of a food like cabbage on acid indi-gestion—with its acid-forming minerals, chlorine, phosphorous, and sulfur notwithstanding—is evidence that foods high in acidic minerals are not the cause of degenerative disease; on the contrary, they have great curative value.

The Preventive Role of Whole Grains

Many studies show that whole grains are an effective remedy for an ulcerated stomach. Where unrefined wheat is the dietary staple, for example, in northern India and China and parts of Africa, ulcers are rare. On the other hand, in Japan, where white rice has replaced the traditional brown rice as a dietary staple, peptic ulcers, once almost unheard of, have become common.[4] No one knows just what fiber does to heal ulcers. One theory is that it reduces gastric enzymes, which the medical establishment claims is the cause of acid reflux and ulcers. If this were the case, eating fiber-rich food would worsen ulcers, for it takes a lot of gastric enzymes to break down the fiber in grain.

The theory that fiber toughens the stomach lining has more merit, since the rough texture of fiber acts as a broom, sweeping away the irritating acidic debris lodged in the lining of the stomach. However, according to Frank I. Tovey, a surgeon and ulcer researcher at the University of London, the fact that ulcers have skyrocketed everywhere in the world since 1900—along with the rise in coronary heart disease—when the removal of the husk covering the grain became widespread, suggests that some of the benefits of fiber come from the nutrients it harbors, particularly vitamins E and B, in addition to the fact that it moves waste matter along the intestinal tract.[5]

Because meat eaters (parasympathetic dominant) don't digest grains well, they have to satisfy most of their fiber requirements with raw fruits and vegetables, which don't have the quantity of B and E vitamins that grains have. This makes vitamin E and a multiple B supplement—preferably in the form of whole-food complexes—a necessity for those with a meat-eating metabolism who suffer from acid indigestion and ulcers.

The Mucilage in Bananas, Plantains, and Cabbage Juice

Bananas and plantains—especially green plantains—and raw cabbage juice heal ulcers by thickening the mucous lining of the stomach. Dr. Ralph Best, a British pharmacist at the University of Aston in Birming-

---

SUGGESTIONS FOR ULCERS*

➤ **Potatoes.** Choose Yukon Gold, cooked lightly to maintain their crunchy texture, and eat once or twice a day with lightly cooked vegetables. The Irish who lived on a diet of potatoes left the skins on when they boiled them and used the water as a base for soup.

➤ **Gelatin.** Use one-half to one ounce in liquid or sprinkled on food three times daily. (See Resources.) This is an excellent source of mucilage.

➤ **Raw vegetables.** Eat with every meal to provide the mucilage and water needed for digestion.

➤ **Raw cabbage juice.** Drink two glasses a day or as much as needed.

➤ **Bananas or plantains.** Eat as many as you comfortably can every day.

➤ **Vitamin E** (400 to 1,600 units/day). Researchers Jon A. Kangas, Ph.D., K. Michael Schmidt, Ph.D., and George F. Solomon, M.D., reported in *The American Journal for Clinical Nutrition* in September 1972 that of two groups of mice subjected to stress, the group given 100 units of vitamin E daily had far fewer and less severe ulcers than the control group.[8]

➤ **Vitamin A** (25,000 to 50,000 units/day). Experiments conducted and written up by T. L. Harris and originally published in the *Society for Experimental Biology and Medicine*, March 1947, show that rats given vitamin A as well as vitamin E had no ulcers at autopsy.[9] Vitamin A helps build mucous membranes.

➤ **Vitamin C** (500 mg/day). In building up collagen, the "glue" that holds the epithelial cells together on the surface of organs, vitamin C helps ensure the integrity of the digestive tract lining.

---

*Take as many as possible of these nutrients in the form of whole-food complexes.

ham, observed a thickening of the stomach wall in autopsies of animals fed banana powder. Dr. Garnett Cheney, a researcher at Stanford University, wrote in the *Journal of the American Dietetic Association* in 1950 of his treatment of twenty-six ulcer patients with cabbage juice, twenty-four of whom made a complete recovery in three to four weeks.[6] Of the nineteen patients in the group treated with conventional medicines, only six recovered. Dr. E. M. Vermel in a Russian medical journal, *Clinical Medicine*, published in 1960, stated that many independent investigations confirmed Dr. Cheney's research and that stomach ulcers disappeared in 85 percent of the 500 subjects in these studies.[7] Vermel believes that vitamin U, about which nothing is known, supplies a nutrient needed for the formation of mucus. I would say, rather, that the factor in bananas and cabbage that rebuilds the stomach's mucous lining is hyaluronic acid, the substance in mucilage that gives it its slippery and gluelike texture.

Despite all the documentation showing the healing effect of cabbage juice and banana powder on ulcers, the treatment of choice for ulcers in recent years has become antibiotics. This is due to the two Australian medical researchers, Doctors Barry Marshall and Robin Warren, who concluded from their research that *H. pylori* bacteria is the cause of ulcers. Their discovery made antibiotics appear to be a cure for ulcers and so obscured the need to find out why the bacteria settled in the stomach in the first place. In fact, bacteria thrive on acidic waste; so they settle wherever acid levels are high, and wherever this is the case the tissue is already inflamed. Inflamed tissue in the stomach and duodenum (uppermost part of the small intestine) is likely to become ulcerated. As bacteria die and the remains turn into acidic waste, inflammation becomes more severe, increasing the likelihood that more ulcers will form. By killing off the *H. pylori* bacteria, antibiotics reduce the inflammation, but they can't eliminate the redness and swelling caused by dietary acidic waste. Only after the foods that triggered the inflammation are no longer eaten can inflamed and ulcerated tissues heal completely.

Gallbladder Problems

It is ironic that a cholesterol-rich saturated fat diet helps prevent gallstones when bile crystallizes into gallstones only when the gallbladder becomes supersaturated with cholesterol. Two siblings, John and Margaret, are examples of what happens when cholesterol is excluded from the diet. Their mother gave them plenty of vegetables, salads, and fruit, but being excessively cholesterol conscious, she served only lean meat and no butter.

Margaret's and John's only source of fatty acids was olive oil in the salads they had every night with their dinner. Both suffered from constipation.

When John graduated from college and moved to his own apartment, he ate out every night at fast-food restaurants where he invariably ordered a cheeseburger and French fries. Nevertheless, from the day he left home his constipation vanished. John was now eating saturated fats, and this change in diet, despite its nutritional deficiencies and chemical additives, had solved his elimination problem. His younger sister, Margaret, however, continued to have the problem after she moved away from home. Like her mother, she avoided butter and trimmed the fat off meat. She also took birth control pills. Five years later she stopped taking them long enough to become pregnant. About a year after she had given birth to a son, she went back on birth control pills. One night she woke up in agony. Pain from a spot under her right rib cage, where the gallbladder is located, radiated into her chest and down her left arm. Afraid that she was having a heart attack, her husband rushed her to the hospital where an MRI revealed gallstones. One of them, half an inch in diameter, was blocking her gallbladder duct. The bile, trapped in the gallbladder by the obstruction, had been diverted into the bloodstream, giving her skin and the whites of her eyes a yellowish tint. Because the gallbladder was badly inflamed, the doctors removed it.

Margaret met three of the criteria that have been linked to gallstones. She had been on a low-cholesterol diet for years, had been constipated for the same period of time, and had been taking birth control pills. A low-cholesterol diet, by causing constipation, can pave the way for gallstones. Cholesterol is one of the raw materials out of which bile salts are made. Bile salts stimulate peristalsis—the alternate contraction and relaxation of the muscles in the intestinal tract that helps overcome elimination problems. Thus a diet low in cholesterol can result in a deficiency of bile salts with the consequent slowing up of the movement of the muscles in the colon, making elimination of stool more difficult.

Constipation increases the likelihood of gallstones by causing the waste matter in the colon to putrefy and give off toxins. If these toxins can't be detoxified by the liver or kidneys, the liver incorporates them in bile. The bile is released into the gallbladder. There, it bonds with cholesterol and hardens into stone. A case control study by F. Pixley, originally published in *Gut*, titled "Dietary Factors in the Etiology of Gallstones," showed a relationship between stone formation and supersaturated quantities of cholesterol in the bladder.[10] Gallstones can also form when the liver and kidneys are too congested to process the fatty acids altered by excessive blood levels of estrogen.

Allergy-causing foods are also a factor in gallbladder attacks and the formation of gallstones. A study carried out by Dr. James C. Breneman back in the 1960s provides evidence for this claim. The 69 patients in his study, all of whom suffered from recurrent gallbladder attacks, were put on an elimination diet to determine their food allergies. Those of the 69 patients who avoided the foods they were allergic to had no more attacks. The primary offending foods were eggs (92.8 percent), pork (63.8 percent), onions (52.2 percent), chicken and turkey (34.8 percent), milk (24.6 percent), coffee (21.7 percent), and oranges (18.8 percent).

JIM'S ALLERGY TO SHELLFISH PRECIPITATED A GALLBLADDER ATTACK

Jim went on a cruise through the Inland Passage to Alaska. He went less to see the fjords and glaciers than for the limitless quantities of food on the buffet table. On the fourth night of the cruise he ate between thirty and forty prawns for dinner. A half hour later he felt a sharp pain in his abdomen. The doctor on board the ship diagnosed a gallbladder attack and blamed it on the huge plate of prawns Jim had eaten. His second attack, which occurred two weeks after the cruise, also occurred after he had eaten prawns.

The pain was so unbearable that his wife rushed him to the hospital where he was given intravenous fluids and was put on a complete fast until the pain went away. It occurred to his wife that since he felt fine once his stomach was emptied of the prawns, and his second attack also occurred after he had eaten prawns, he might be having an allergic reaction to the prawns. Jim's doctor disagreed. He didn't see how a food allergy could cause the gallbladder to malfunction. Convinced that allergy tests would be a waste of time, he told Jim that with his gallbladder removed he could eat all the prawns he wanted.

continued

But after the operation Jim continued to experience symptoms of gallbladder trouble and, contrary to the doctor's prediction, especially after he ate prawns!

Jim finally agreed to have allergy tests, which confirmed his wife's contention that he was allergic to shellfish. But now in addition to a problem with prawns, he gets an upset stomach whenever he eats butter or olive oil—not an unusual aftermath of gallbladder surgery. The reason is that the liver interprets the gallbladder's disappearance to mean that it no longer needs to produce a large amount of bile. As a result, in those who have their gallbladder removed, fats and oils are only partially digested.

SUGGESTIONS FOR GALLSTONES

➤ **Grapes, beets, and endive.** These foods detoxify the liver, kidneys, and gallbladder and improve digestion and elimination.

➤ **Ice pack.** The cold relieves pain during a gallbladder attack by reducing inflammation.

➤ **Whole grains (if you have a grain-eating metabolism).** These provide roughage and vitamins B and E. Manna bread, made with sprouted seeds, provides food enzymes in addition to the nutrients found in whole-grain bread.

➤ **Thyroid medication.** An underactive thyroid can reduce the secretion of gastric juice in the stomach and has been linked to gallbladder disease. If tests indicate an underactive thyroid, have your progesterone checked to see if your progesterone level is low. Natural progesterone supplements, by increasing progesterone levels, normalize thyroid function.

➤ **Cayenne pepper.** Cayenne stimulates good digestion, including the breakdown of fats, which helps prevent gallstones without irritating the stomach. (It's also a good overall body tonic. The West Indians in Jamaica, where the cayenne plant grows in profusion on the sides of mountains, nibble on a cayenne leaf whenever they feel sick because its healing properties reach out to all illnesses.)

➤ **Ox bile.** Take two capsules with meals. When there isn't enough bile because some of it has crystallized into gallstones or the gallbladder has been removed, ox bile is a good substitute. (See Resources.)

➤ **Lipase.** Two capsules with each meal will help bile emulsify fats.

➤ **Olive oil.** Three to four tablespoons a day increase the flow of bile.

➤ **The gallbladder flush.** Drink as much apple juice as possible for three or four days. (The malic acid in apples helps dissolve gallstones.) On the fifth, sixth, and seventh day, use a castor oil pack on the liver for one hour. On the eighth day, take two teaspoons of Epsom salts after lunch, and two hours later take two more teaspoons of Epsom salts. On day nine eat only a grapefruit for dinner, and at bedtime drink four ounces of extra-virgin olive oil. Sleep on your right side. The next morning, one hour before breakfast, take two teaspoons of Epsom salts.

➤ **Vitamins.** See the supplement suggestions at the end of the section on ulcers.

➤ **Ground psyllium husks and clay.** When suspended in water mixed in juice these are good colon cleansers.

Allergy-causing foods most likely trigger gallbladder attacks in this way: The digestive enzymes receive a signal from the immune cells that the food is a foreign substance, so they stay way from it. As a result, the food remains undigested and degenerates into acidic waste. When acidic waste level reaches a critical point, it flows into the small intestine and from there through the bile duct to the gallbladder. Once in the gallbladder it becomes raw material for the formation of gallstones. It also irritates the gallbladder, which becomes disoriented and directs the flow of the bile to the wrong organ. Instead of going into the small intestine from the gallbladder where it breaks down fat, the bile flows into the stomach where it interferes with digestion by neutralizing hydrochloric acid, the substance that digests protein.

Colitis, Ileitis, and Other Inflammatory Intestinal Disorders

Bess, age sixty-six, had had colitis (inflammation of the colon) and ileitis (inflammation of the section of the small intestine that joins the colon) since her midtwenties. Like many individuals with an inflammatory intestinal condition, she had mental problems. It was an attribute she had inherited; many members of her family suffered from depression, several had committed suicide, and three of her grandparents had died of Alzheimer's disease. Bess's anxiety led to feelings of depression so severe that they clouded over the sunny disposition she had had as a child. She came to hate herself, not just who she was but the way she looked. For twenty years she had avoided looking at herself in the mirror. The little self-esteem she possessed went into her nails, which she kept beautifully manicured. Despite all her insecurities, she charmed everyone she met and was extremely well informed on almost any topic that came up in a conversation.

Bess had been something of a child prodigy. She learned to read at the age of eighteen months and was reading a newspaper at the age of two. She has a talent similar to those of idiot savants. Without looking, she can write at the same time with both hands, her left hand writing from left to right and her right hand from right to left until her hands meet.

The most recent of Bess's colitis and ileitis attacks had occurred when she removed books from the bookshelves in her living room so they could be painted. Looking at the empty bookshelves triggered painful cramps, bloating, and diarrhea. After the shelves had been painted and the books replaced, she had an even worse attack of cramps and diarrhea. Bess had had so many bouts of diarrhea over the years that she had developed ulcerated colitis. Her inflammatory bowel disorders were synchronized with her attacks of anxiety.

Not all individuals with inflammatory intestinal problems experience the same severe stress levels as Bess, but it's hard to find anyone with this disorder who doesn't insist that it is triggered by anxiety. The stress might be the result of a major upheaval such as being fired from a job or the death of a close relative, but more likely it arises from taking on a responsibility that isn't part of the daily routine: redoing a kitchen, planning a wedding, job hunting, making preparations for a trip, working overtime, and so on.

The Worsening of an Intestinal Problem Because of an Environmental Pollutant

Maria tells the story of standing in the doorway of her son Foster's bedroom one morning, when, as he woke up, he looked at her and remarked that she had just cleaned her teeth. He said he could smell the mint flavor of her toothpaste—despite the fact that Maria hadn't opened her mouth even to say good morning. Foster had developed this acute sense of smell after he and his family moved into a house that, unbeknownst to them at the time, harbored toxic mold.

Foster had had an intestinal yeast infection since he was a baby. The fact that his stool had turned yellow after moving into the tainted house indicated his yeast infection had worsened. With the multiplication of the yeast cells accelerating, more yeast cells were dying off and turning into acid waste. This additional acid waste increased his already-elevated blood acid levels, which, in turn, raised his stress-promoting hormone levels. These raised levels increased Foster's anxiety and depression.

Foster and his family have moved out of the toxic house, but he is still battling his intestinal yeast infection and accompanying emotional problems.

The intestines are far more vulnerable to injury from acid waste than the stomach because they don't have the thick mucous lining the stomach has. (The thin mucous lining in the intestines enables digested food to pass through the intestinal walls into the blood and lymph circulatory systems.) Acidic waste injures the intestines in several ways. Besides inflaming intestinal tissues, it kills off the friendly bacteria that aid in digestion and extract nutrients from digesting food. Diarrhea is one outcome. The other is that invading microorganisms are no longer kept in check. These unfriendly germs give off such poisonous wastes as alcohol, ammonia, acetaldehyde, and formaldehyde, which, when elevated, destroy the intestines' mucous lining. Once this protective barrier is gone, the toxins make scratches, tears, and holes in the intestinal walls and, along with sharp acidic particles, wear away the lining of the colon, thinning it out until it is stretched so tight that it balloons out and forms sacs (diverticula) in which waste matter gets lodged.

Appendectomy

There are other causes of intestinal inflammation besides mental stress. One is the removal of the appendix. This operation, from 1900 to around 1950, was almost as common as tonsillectomy. The justification for its removal was that it was a vestigial (useless) organ. That in fact the appendix has a vital function in the body is suggested by several studies that have correlated appendectomies with an increase in cancer. A study of 1,165 patients at the Medical College in Toledo, Ohio, conducted by Dr. George Padanilam showed that 67 percent of the patients who had developed cancer before the age of fifty had had their appendix removed;[11] and Dr. Howard Bierman of the Institute for Cancer and Blood Research, speaking at the American College of Surgeons in 1966, said that according to his studies, out of hundreds of cancer patients, 84 percent had had their appendixes removed whereas only 25 percent of the noncancer patients were missing their appendixes.[12]

These studies make a strong case that the appendix, like the tonsils and adenoids, is part of the immune system and as such produces antibodies that not only destroy cancer-causing viruses but also engulf and dispose of the toxins and bacteria that inflame the bowels. The appendix's location at the bottom of the ascending colon clearly indicates that its purpose is to protect the small intestine from the toxic waste in the ascending colon.

According to Michael Crichton, M.D., in his book *Five Patients*, appendix operations started with the pathologist Reginald H. Fitz's assertion that inflammation, pus, and pain in the lower right abdomen was caused by an infection in the appendix.[13] This hypothesis, Crichton writes, created a new disease. Although many physicians resisted the idea of removing the appendix, eventually the surgeons won out. The final victory for the appendix removal proponents was achieved in 1902 when England's King Edward VII had an appendectomy. Shortly afterward, the operation came into vogue. Physicians were not then aware, as most still aren't today, that inflammation from toxic acidic waste is the initial cause of appendicitis. (In China today hospitals typically offer patients with appendicitis two choices: an appendectomy or a program of herbs and diet to detoxify the appendix, thus avoiding the necessity for an operation.)

Other Causes of Inflammatory Intestinal Disorders

Doctors no longer remove the appendix as a matter of course, but this hasn't decreased inflammatory bowel disease, because new medical interventions have come into use that are damaging to the intestinal tract. Irritable bowel syndrome, Crohn's disease, and colitis became commonplace when antibiotics came into widespread use more than fifty years ago. Bacteria that survive antibiotic treatment develop a resistance to it, possibly by producing a virulent toxin that destroys the antibiotics—and also damages the intestinal walls. The measles vaccination has also increased bowel disease. A British study of 3,545 individuals who received measles vaccinations showed that there was a threefold increase in Crohn's disease and a two-and-a-half-fold increase in ulcerative colitis as compared to a control group.[14] The formaldehyde, mercury, and diseased animal tissue in vaccines all contribute to the breakdown of intestinal tissues.

The results of a Swedish study shows a relationship between junk food and an increase in intestinal disorders that is hardly surprising.[15] According to the study, those who eat fast foods at least twice a week are 3.4 times more likely to develop Crohn's disease and 3.9 times more likely to develop ulcerative colitis. Junk food debris, like antibiotics, vaccines, and mental stress, produces acidic waste that triggers the flow of adrenal hormones. These hormones divert the flow of blood from the digestive tract to the cardiovascular system, the first step in the march toward inflammatory bowel disease.

Curing Inflammatory Intestinal Disorders

Bowel disorders can be relieved by reducing stress. When the calming effect is achieved, the two halves of the autonomic nervous system—the sympathetic and parasympathetic nerves—become better balanced. This balance brings on a more even distribution of the blood and lymph fluids, so that all the organ systems receive their fair share of nutrients and oxygen. This in turn improves digestion and the transit of food and waste through the digestive tract, which gives the intestines a chance to heal.

Bess healed her colitis and ileitis by relieving her anxiety and depression. She took a supplement called SAM-e. (SAM-e is activated methionine.) SAM-e increases the production of the neurotransmitters that have a calming effect and lower stress hormone levels—L-dopa, dopamine, and phosphatidylcholine. Bess also took Aangamik, which relieves depression by oxygenating the brain cells. After she had been on this regimen for several months, she no longer felt anxious over the least deviation in her daily routine, and her feelings of depression lifted. She was the first member of her family to have conquered a mental disorder. Her calmness indicated that her stress-promoting hormone levels had dropped. The resulting increase in blood flow to the intestines normalized her intestinal function.

A major cause of intestinal disorders is bad diet, which is most likely a contributing factor in cases where mental stress is the primary cause. Anyone with a bowel disorder should try to reduce intestinal inflammation by avoiding foods that produce an allergic reaction and by eating only organically grown foods based on their metabolic type. Martha's intestinal function got better when she made some changes in her diet. She tested herself for food allergies (see Chapter 2) and found that she was lactose intolerant, the most common allergy in people with intestinal inflammation. (In a study of 77 patients with irritable bowel syndrome conducted by Italian physicians, 74 percent were found to be allergic to milk. They were put on a milk-free diet for three weeks, and their condition in all cases improved.[16]) Martha's attacks of diarrhea became less frequent but didn't go away entirely, so she took three tablespoons of bran three times a day to strengthen the intestinal walls. Eating bran on a regular basis speeds up the transit time of stool by increasing peristaltic movement. In Martha's case, however, it acted as an irritant, causing her intestines to become more inflamed. Discouraged, she went to her family doctor for treatment. He told her that raw garlic was effective for all forms of inflammatory bowel disease but asked her to keep it confidential—what if it got around that he had recommended a folk remedy! It always worked, he said. The patient had to eat as many raw cloves of garlic as he or she could stand, fixed in a variety of different ways to make it more palatable. Martha tried the garlic remedy, and it worked just as her doctor said it would.

John started having digestive problems when he was twenty. By the time he was thirty-five he had developed Crohn's disease, an extremely severe inflammatory bowel disorder. He tried to avoid foods that gave him indigestion, but his job took him all over the world, and his digestive tract couldn't adjust to foods that differed from one country to the next. His intestines became so inflamed that the doctor prescribed prednisone, a steroid hormone. When that didn't work, he had three feet of his intestines and his ileocaecal valve removed. Fearing that if his inflamed bowel condition continued to worsen he would end up with no intestines at all, John began investigating alternative remedies. I suggested castor oil, the best remedy for a sluggish gut and one that has been used for many ailments since biblical times. The oil is extracted from the castor bean, which grows on a tree called the Palma Christi. According to Edgar Cayce, castor oil activates peristalsis in the colon by triggering a chemical action in which water splits oil into glycerol and the fatty acid ricinoleic acid.

John placed a castor oil pack on his lower abdomen for one hour every day for one week and took one tablespoon of the oil every morning before breakfast. In a week his stools, which had been either too loose or too hard, assumed a normal consistency. His abdominal cramps and pain, however, hadn't gone away because his intestines were still inflamed, a sign that his bowel was still hyperacidic. To increase the alkalinity of his intestines, John slept on a far infrared pad (see Resources). He also drank alkaline water. A month later he broke out in a rash and had open, running sores all over his abdomen. The acidic waste in his gut had been dissolved and excreted through the skin. With this removal, the pain and inflammation in John's intestinal tract vanished.

As the personal stories in this chapter reveal, the way to cure digestive tract problems is to neutralize the acid wastes in the body. While this can be done with alkaline-based products such as the infrared mat and alkaline water, clearly the most effective treatment is an allergy-free diet that takes into consideration an individual's metabolic type—meat eater, grain eater, or the balanced metabolism.

SUGGESTIONS FOR INFLAMMATORY
INTESTINAL DISORDERS*

➤ **Far infrared pad.** This pad alkalinizes the intestinal tract.

➤ **Melatonin.** Melatonin reduces stress hormone levels. Start with 0.3 mg and increase the dosage until the desired effect is obtained. Maximum dosage is 5 mg. (Do not take melatonin if you have an autoimmune disease.)

➤ **SAM-e** (200 to 600 mg/day). This supplement lowers stress hormone levels by improving brain function.

➤ **Aangamik.** Aangamik relieves the stress caused by depression by oxygenating the brain. Follow directions on the box.

➤ **Caprylic acid** (365 mg/day). You will need two tablets. It destroys yeast cells in the intestinal tract.

➤ **Garlic.** Have as much as you can eat for two to three days, preferably raw. Raw garlic clears up inflammation in the intestinal tract. Proceed with care if the intestinal walls are severely lacerated.

➤ **Castor oil packs.** Place on lower abdomen for one hour a day for a minimum of one week.

➤ **Castor oil.** Take one to two tablespoons. Castor oil relieves constipation by activating peristaltic movement in the intestines.

➤ **Ice pack.** Whenever the abdomen feels hot as a result of inflammation, an ice pack lessons the redness and swelling.

➤ **Slippery elm tea.** Drink it warm, not hot.

➤ **Vitamin E** (400 to 800 units/day). As a cancer preventative, vitamin E also heals hemorrhoids, which are caused more often by inappropriate diet than are any other intestinal inflammatory conditions.

➤ **Multiple vitamin and mineral supplements.** Take these to replace the nutrients that in intestinal disease often don't get absorbed into the bloodstream.

➤ **Acupuncture.** It helps normalize blood circulation.

➤ **Pureed carrots.** This remedy is good for diarrhea, especially in babies and small children.

*Take as many as possible of these nutrients in the form of whole-food complexes. Follow the directions on the label.

CHAPTER 4

OBESITY

M y colleagues and I were sitting around a table in the faculty lounge of the university where we teach, discussing the untimely death of Jim, an administrator, from a stroke. Only forty-eight years old, he was sixty to seventy-five pounds overweight and had high blood pressure. Because of his craving for junk food he hadn't followed his doctor's advice to go on a calorie-reducing diet. One colleague quoted a United States government survey that showed that in 2008, eight out of ten individuals over the age of twenty-five are overweight. Being grossly overweight, defined as fifty pounds over the norm based on height, is linked to every major degenerative disease, including cancer, heart disease, diabetes, and arthritis.

A diet suited to the individual's metabolic type is especially important for those who are fifty or more pounds overweight, for the excess acid waste from a metabolically inappropriate diet in those who are obese is converted by the body into fatty acid and stored in fat molecules in the body. Thus it is not only excess calories that put on weight but also undigested food that acidifies.

Raw Foods Prevent Excessive Weight Gain

We should emulate, to the extent possible, the raw food–eating habits of preindustrial cultures, because for nearly all of the three hundred thousand years of protohuman's existence, everything was eaten raw. It was only with the Wurm Glacial period sixty-five thousand years ago

HOW THE ASHANTI KEEP SLIM

Was it possible, I asked my colleagues, for a group of people on earth to remain insulated from the kind of chemicalized, processed food that had spawned the obesity epidemic in the United States? One professor, who came from Ghana, West Africa, said that the Ashanti of Ghana were one such people. He said they were the envy of neighboring tribes because of their slim, willowy figures. He had been told by non-Ashanti Ghanans that there were no fat Ashanti because they ate such huge quantities of plantains.

In fact, the plantain is just one of many foods that explain why the Ashanti are not obese. The slimming effect of the Ashanti diet is assured by the fact that, like their ancestors, many of them still obtain their food by trapping and foraging.

The Neolithic era, characterized by a planned economy and cultivation of the soil, had passed the Ashanti by, because the territory of the Ashanti is forested. In the forest there is no grassy savanna for cattle to graze on and no sunlit fields for planting grains, so farming and herding are impossible. Instead, the Ashanti trap small animals and deer, fish in streams, dig up such root vegetables as wild yam and cassava, and pick plantains off trees. Nothing that grows in the tangled vines, swamps, and dense foliage of the forest floor has been enriched and fattened by humans. The nutritional content of these wild foodstuffs is enough for the Ashanti's energy and the repair and regeneration of their body tissues, but it is not enough to make them fat.

that humans began cooking with fire, thus destroying the enzymes in foods that prevent obesity. Enzymes keep weight down, because, like workers at a construction site who use just enough bricks and mortar to put a building together, they convert the food we eat into the exact quantity of raw materials needed for maintaining and rebuilding the body. The rest is eliminated.

However, in the case of enzyme-free cooked food, there is nothing to prevent too many nutrients from being absorbed into the body's cells. What the body doesn't need is stored in fat cells located in loose connective (adipose) tissue. Cooked food also causes weight gain because, taking longer to digest, it leaves food particles behind. Leftover food turns into acidic waste, some of which is stored in the body as fat.

Dr. Edward Howell, in his excellent book *Enzyme Nutrition*, writes that unlike raw food, cooked food stimulates the endocrine glands, causing them to secrete excessive levels of hormones.[1] This increases body weight because hormones regulate body functions. They switch body functions on and off according to the body's needs. An excessive level of hormones turns the production centers in the cells on too often, causing the over-production of nutrients. Excess nutrients are stored in fat molecules under the skin. A study in which the effects on weight gain between canned and raw food are compared supports Howell's contention. Conducted by E. F. Kohman, W. H. Eddy, Mary E. White, and N. H. Sanborn of Columbia University and published in *The Journal of Nutrition* in 1977, the study concluded that canned food, which must be cooked at a high temperature, caused more weight gain than the same food left raw.[2]

Monosodium glutamate (MSG), which is added to many bottled and canned foods as well as poultry and fast foods, is also linked to weight gain. A review of the article "Diabetes Danger in a Taste of Chinese" states that scientists have discovered that MSG affects insulin secretion.[3] Since MSG is known to excite the endocrine glands, it is safe to conclude that the beta cells in the pancreas that produce insulin, when exposed to MSG, become whipped up and overproduce it. Excessive levels of insulin lower blood sugar excessively. The resulting low blood sugar, referred to as hypoglycemia, is associated with obesity, probably because the excess glucose that is removed from the blood is converted to fat. Elevated insulin is not only associated with obesity but also with the recurrence of breast cancer. It can be lowered by taking pantothenic acid, a B vitamin. (Specific suggestions are given at the end of this chapter.)

MSG is not the only artificial chemical that promotes obesity. Any foods that are altered by chemical additives confuse the appestat mechanism. This is the part of the brain that signals us to eat when our stomachs are empty and our body tissues need nourishment by creating hunger pangs. It tells us to stop when our stomachs are full and nutrient requirements are met, by creating a feeling of satiety. Chemicalized foods tend to stimulate hunger, even when the body does not need nutrients. Another factor contributing to obesity is eating food deficient in such alkaline minerals as calcium, magnesium, and potassium. (This includes most processed foods.) Alkaline minerals are needed to neutralize the acidic waste that is the by-product of even the most nutritious foods. When the supply of alkaline minerals is low, acidic wastes don't get neutralized. While some of the fatty acids in the waste are stored as body fat, other fatty acids are converted to cholesterol and lactic acid. This increases the acid levels in the blood and lymph fluids, which makes the body more vulnerable to weight gain because as blood, loaded with acidic waste, circulates, it clogs organ systems. This slows down metabolism so that correspondingly less food (fuel) is burned up.

Excessive weight gain is also caused by the consumption of refined grains. Even before our digestive enzyme glands had a chance to adjust to the kind and quantity of enzymes needed to break down the grains that had been introduced into the diet only around seven thousand years ago, manufacturers (in the early 1900s) started tampering with them by removing the husks.

The health benefits of whole grains are not just in the nutritional content. They take longer to digest than refined grains. The advantage of slow digestion is that blood sugar levels don't rise excessively. Refined grains, on the other hand, are broken down so quickly they leave behind excessive levels of glucose in the blood. This is another case where high blood sugar levels are converted by insulin to fat.

Excessive glucose in the liver is converted to fat just as it is in the blood. A fatty liver is more dangerous to health than layers of fat under the skin because the fat globules in the liver prevent it from detoxifying digested food plus performing its myriad other functions.

What's Wrong with a High-Protein, Low-Carbohydrate Diet?

Many people who want to lose weight look for the silver bullet that doesn't demand too much sacrifice but still guarantees weight loss. This is usually a diet that prohibits some foods while allowing unrestricted consumption of others. For example, one diet that was popular in the 1950s was all the bananas and ice cream you could eat but nothing else. This was a one-week diet. Another allows hardly any fat but the unrestricted consumption of carbohydrates. Such diets are appealing because they promise relief from ravenous hunger by allowing the dieter to pig out on one or two foods.

The most popular diet since it first appeared in England in 1860, in William Banting's book, *Letter on Corpulence*, and more recently in Dr.

Robert C. Atkins's *New Diet Revolution*, is the high-protein, high-fat, low-carbohydrate diet. Its popularity is understandable because it takes weight off relatively easily, and eating lots of meats seems to lessen the hunger pangs that drive many people to binge eating—at least in the beginning.

But if the objective in losing weight is to improve health, that should be the driving force behind the choice of diet. The high-protein, low-carbohydrate diet does not fulfill that objective, because it is unbalanced. Eating so little starch deprives the body of glucose, its primary source of fuel, while eating too much meat threatens the body's mineral reserves. Excessive phosphate levels in meat can remove calcium and magnesium from the teeth and bones. Another danger to the body's supply of alkaline minerals is blood nitrogen urea from the breakdown of meat. Too much meat in the diet produces excessively high urea levels that the kidneys excrete along with magnesium and calcium.

Shifting viewpoints of the medical establishment as to what constitutes a healthy meal, as well as trendiness in diets, has made us lose sight of what used to be the axiom of nutritionists and doctors: the balanced meal made up of meat, potatoes, vegetables, and a lettuce and tomato salad. Indigenous cultures were not so quick to forget the knowledge of good nutrition passed on to them by their ancestors.

In most tribal societies in Africa, including both meat and starches in every meal was a time-honored tradition because it reflected the social structure of the clan. For example, among the Kaguru of central Tanzania a meal was said to be made up of both *ugali* (starches such as maize, millet, rice, plantain, and cassava) and *nyama* (stew meat). Only when nyama was not available did *mboga* (vegetables) take its place. Ugali represented the feminine gender because it was cultivated by women, while nyama was masculine because it was obtained by men's work as herdsmen and hunters. The well-balanced diets of these preindustrial cultures prevented obesity because they did not produce excessive levels of fatty acid wastes that build up layers of fat in the body.

Fighting Obesity with Acid-Alkaline Balance

The morbidly obese have unbalanced biochemistry. For many in this category hunger is not satisfied even when the stomach is filled. There are people who fall into the morbidly obese category even though they are moderate eaters.

Cheryl fit into the latter category. She was seventeen years old at the time I met her, weighed 350 pounds, and was five feet, six inches tall. Cheryl's mother showed me her medical records. Physical examinations by an endocrinologist, which included blood tests every year since she was twelve, failed to show any abnormalities in glandular function, blood lipid levels, or blood pressure. Nevertheless, Cheryl had some symptoms of ill health such as migraine headaches, depression, and swollen ankles and feet.

A ravenous appetite, however, was not one of her problems. At times she went all day without eating because she wasn't hungry. Her one liking was for sweets, and she ate two chocolate candy bars at a time once or twice a week, hardly enough to account for being two hundred pounds overweight. I believed Cheryl when she said she was not addicted to sweets, because the favorite marzipan cake her mother made her for her seventeenth birthday was practically intact one week later. Considering the small quantities of food Cheryl ate—her mother actually worried because she was hardly ever hungry—it was obvious she was not burning up her excess body fat. Her body shape was partly responsible. She had been chubby as a little girl, but before adolescence the fat was concentrated around her hips and thighs. As she put on the pounds, the fat crept up into her abdomen and chest. Excess fat in these regions is broken down and released into the bloodstream more quickly than the fat in the lower part of the body. This can lead to heart disease and liver damage.

It was essential for the sake of her health that Cheryl take off the excess layers of fat around the chest and abdomen. At my suggestion, she placed three five-by-twelve-inch magnetic pads over her chest and abdomen at night when she went to bed. Magnetic energy is a useful adjunct in a weight-loss program, because the negative charge of the magnets helps the growth hormone pull fat out of the fat cells. Happily, the removed fat is not deposited elsewhere. Not only do the chest and abdomen areas flatten out, weight typically drops by fifteen to twenty pounds. After about two months Cheryl's chest and upper abdomen were protruding less and she had taken off ten pounds.

Cheryl's rotund shape was not only dangerous to her health; it also made it very difficult for her to burn up fat. To generate additional energy for the purpose of losing weight, she took two teaspoons of coconut oil a day. At room temperature the oil is a solid, white block because it is supersaturated, but unlike meat and some dairy fats, coconut oil is not converted into cholesterol. Nor does it add to the stores of body fat. Being made up of medium chains of fatty acids, it gets burned up quickly. At the end of three months Cheryl had lost twenty pounds. This weight loss seems insignificant in relation to Cheryl's total weight, but it reduced the swelling in her ankles and feet.

To further raise Cheryl's energy level, with her doctor's approval I had her take some thyroid extract even though her thyroid function tested normal. The thyroid supplement raised her body temperature slightly above the normal 98.6 degrees. This caused her body to produce more energy than normal, and she burned off twenty more pounds of fat.

An increase in the production of energy is not much benefit if it isn't transported to wherever it is needed in the body, so Cheryl took 50 mg of CoQ-10 twice a day. But CoQ-10 did not cause further weight loss, probably because Cheryl's energy distribution system was normal. Cheryl melted away another fifteen pounds after she started playing badminton with her father for two hours, three times a week.

The weight that Cheryl lost as a result of these measures alleviated most of her health problems. While she still has migraine headaches, she no longer gets a blind spot in the center of her visual field during an attack, and her depressed moods occur less often. Cheryl's weight stabilized around 220 pounds—not enough weight loss for her to leave the morbidly obese category behind, but enough to make her feel—and look—much better. That was two years ago. Cheryl has maintained her weight loss.

A Scientifically Proven Way to Lose Weight

Most people aren't aware that there is such a thing as brown fat. Brown fat differs from white fat, the fat we are familiar with. While white fat is stored in fat cells, brown fat is burned off by heat. Thus while white fat, in excess, makes us overweight, brown fat, being burned up, would make us slim—if we only had some in our bodies! Since babies have a lot of brown fat, it was assumed that its purpose was to keep their bodies warm. For this reason, medical scientists had assumed adults had no brown fat. Then in April of 2009, Dr. Enerback at the University of Goteburg in Sweden reported that he had found some brown fat tissue in adults.

In the meantime, Dr. Bruce M. Spiegelman of Harvard Medical School discovered the key element in the production of brown fat cells in the body: a protein called zinc fingers.[4] Spiegelman reasoned that if he inactivated this protein in the brown fat cells, they should turn back into what they were before they became brown fat cells—white fat cells. But he had made the wrong assumption, for the brown fat cells didn't revert back to white fat cells upon deactivation of the protein. Instead, they turned into muscle cells.

Spiegelman is now implanting mice with brown fat cells in the hope they will slim the mice down. He won't say how the experiment is going, but he does say that so far the results are encouraging. He hopes to do the same with humans. Because brown fat cells induce the body's white fat cells to break down into fatty acids and then absorbs them, he believes that brown cells inserted in humans will melt off the pounds.

Additional Factors to Consider on a Weight-Loss Diet

What can be done about food addictions? Eating one medium-sized, sliced-up raw potato a day can reduce the craving for food. But there are other alternatives. Cheryl chose one of them. She gave up all the foods she was addicted to at once to see if there were any she could do without. Whereas her craving for pizza and hero sandwiches persisted, she didn't miss sodas. In place of soda, she drinks carbonated water.

One hard-and-fast rule all dieters should follow is no junk food before breakfast. A junk-food snack first thing in the morning ferments and putrefies in the stomach. Any healthy food eaten afterward, exposed to the bacteria in the putrefying and fermenting junk-food molecules, is also broken down into toxic waste by these bacteria.

The most critical factor in any weight-loss program is the efficient digestion of foods. Complete digestion means fewer acidic wastes. This has at least three advantages:

- Appetite cravings are reduced (toxic acidic food residues create abnormal hunger pangs).
- Fewer acidic wastes means less fat sticks to the ribs.
- Reduction in toxic acidic wastes makes for a more alkaline environment in the body. This in turn increases the production of food-digesting enzymes.

Keep in mind that the more enzymes that break down food molecules in the gastrointestinal tract, the less food remains undigested and the better the chances to attain the ultimate in efficient digestion and consequent weight loss: oxidation (burning) of 97 percent of the food you eat.

RAW OR NEARLY RAW POTATOES: LOSE THE DESIRE TO BINGE

When I went on the semiraw potato diet (see Chapter 3) it had an unexpected benefit. It eliminated my intense craving for food. A faster way of eliminating intense food cravings is to eat a few slices of raw potato a day. This can smooth the rough edges off of an intense craving for food in a matter of days.

When the potato diet caused my appetite to diminish it got me to thinking. Potatoes, being highly alkaline, especially when they aren't cooked to death, neutralize acidity. I had been hyperacidic—that's why the potato diet worked so well for me. Then it came to me why this was so. My food binges began at the age of ten. Before that, ear, throat, and stomach infections and three bouts of scarlet fever had killed my appetite, causing such a severe calcium deficiency that I got rickets. The day my childhood illnesses came to an end my appetite switched on. Ten years of continual infections had to have left behind an enormous amount of acid waste from the dead bacteria that had caused my illnesses. This acid waste stimulated my appetite as soon as I stopped getting infections.

SUGGESTIONS FOR WEIGHT LOSS*

➤ **Pantothenic acid** (500 mg/day). Take pantothenic acid to lower elevated insulin levels, common in people who are overweight. Excessive insulin levels are associated with cancer, specifically the recurrence of breast cancer.

➤ **Nearly raw potatoes.** These are effective in reducing hunger pangs. For directions, see Chapter 3.

➤ **Ice pack.** Placed on the lower abdomen, it takes away the appetite.

➤ **Raw milk and butter.** These are worth tracking down because of their rich supply of the fat-digesting enzyme lipase and the enzyme protease for the breakdown of protein. The greater the intake of enzymes the more efficient the digestion, which means less fat is deposited in the fat cells.

continued

➤ **Raw beefsteak.** If the steer have been raised on hormone- and pesticide-free feed, raw beefsteak is a good diet food because it's loaded with protein- and fat-digesting enzymes. Bartenders recommend rare roast beef sandwiches for hangovers because the enzymes in the beef eliminate acid aldehyde, the poisonous by-product of alcohol, which causes the symptoms described as a hangover.

➤ **Avocados and bananas.** These are filling, but when eaten raw they don't cause unnecessary weight gain, and they contain more enzymes than other fruits and vegetables that have fewer calories.

➤ **Vitamin E** (400 mg/day). Not only does vitamin E help normalize thyroid function, it also neutralizes the poisonous by-products of polyunsaturated oils, which interfere with thyroid function. Lowered thyroid production of thyroxin means less heat energy, so less fat is burned up.

➤ **Coconut and flaxseed oil.** Two teaspoons daily help increase energy production.

➤ **Raw carrots.** These remove fat molecules from the body.

➤ **Acidic foods.** Sour-tasting foods such as grape juice, vinegar, and yogurt reduce cravings.

➤ **Bland foods.** They don't excite the taste buds and stimulate hunger.

➤ **Several small meals.** Eating small amounts of food often, rather than three big meals a day, keeps the digestive process working and burning up energy.

➤ **Blackstrap-lemon drink.** Detoxifying the liver is an aid to weight loss because the detoxifying process gets rid of acidic waste. Add two heaping tablespoons of blackstrap molasses and the juice of a lemon to a glass of hot water. Drink nothing but this concoction for three days. Sip it slowly. Repeat this procedure every few months.

➤ **Ice water.** Drink a glass of it before a meal. This reduces weight because in order to maintain the body's internal temperature, which has dropped due to the cold water, the body burns up additional calories.

*Take as many of these supplements as possible in the form of whole-food complexes. Follow the directions on the label.

CHAPTER 5

THYROID PROBLEMS

Sunlight is the stimulus that makes it possible for the thyroid to regulate the production of energy in the body. The stage is set for this assembly-line process when the first rays of sunlight in the morning are absorbed into the pigment of the brain's pineal gland. This act signals the pineal—the regulator of the sleeping-waking cycle of the body—to pass on the message via the pituitary gland to the thyroid that it must release additional thyroxin (T4) for the production of more energy. T4 flows through the bloodstream to the cells and delivers the message. (Before T4 can deliver this message, it must be converted by the liver into T3.) With the increased flow of energy to the organ systems, their functions speed up. This enables man to begin his daily struggle for existence.

The many diseases associated with deficient energy—cancer, hardening of the arteries, arthritis, diabetes, and obesity—make clear that a lack of energy because of a low-functioning thyroid can cut short our struggle for existence while we are still in our prime. Until I reached middle age, I was unaware that my illnesses were symptoms of energy levels so low that they couldn't sustain normal body function. I was lacking in energy even as an infant. I didn't walk until eighteen months and didn't start talking until the age of three, at which time I began getting very painful canker sores—another symptom of hypothyroidism. My slowness was attributed to the "lazy baby" syndrome and the canker sores to an allergy to oranges.

By the time I was thirty, my eyes had become oversensitive to light. Even in winter on a gray day I wore sunglasses and left them on when entering a store because of the glare from the fluorescent lights. During the winter I caught one viral infection after another. Each infection lasted for two weeks, and my canker sores had become so painful they kept me in bed for days.

In trying to heal myself, I ignored the role of the thyroid in regulating the energy needs of the body—until treating each symptom separately no longer worked. Like a mechanic who repairs first one broken-down part of a car and then another, I had treated each malfunctioning organ as a separate entity. Now I took the reverse approach. I recognized that all my health problems were due to a single cause: low thyroid function.

I took the basal thermometer test, a method for testing thyroid function discovered by Dr. Broda Barrens. Hundreds of studies in England have verified that this test is a far more reliable measurement of an underactive thyroid than testing the thyroid stimulating hormone (TSH) blood levels.[1] My waking temperature, which was 96.1, confirmed that I had extremely low thyroid function. A blood test, showing my TSH blood level to be 20   far too high—thus confirmed my depressed thyroid function as revealed by my low body temperature.

I took thyroid medication, first synthroid and then thyroxin, for more than a year but developed allergic reactions to both medications. They made me feel restless, and my hair stood on end as though an electric current were running through it. Once I went off all thyroid medications, my thyroid symptoms returned. I was frightened until an idea out of the blue struck me: maybe my depressed thyroid was caused by an allergic reaction to certain foods. Aware that the foods and/or beverages consumed most often are the offending allergens, I reduced the number of cups of tea I drank every day from fifteen to one. Since then I have not been plagued by canker sores, fatigue, viral infections, or eye sensitivity. Confirming that an allergy to tea was the cause of my slow thyroid was the fact that my below-normal basal temperature had gone up to 98.5. The irony is that although a slow thyroid was undoubtedly at the root of my "lazy baby" syndrome, my thyroid must have normalized by the time I became an adult but then was being "held down" by my overconsumption of tea.

Testing for Underactive Thyroid

The basal thermometer test is a good way to start measuring your thyroid activity. Take your temperature with an old-fashioned mercury thermometer. It's the only reliable thermometer device. Place under the tongue or under your arm for seven to ten minutes three or four times a day. Upon waking before you get out of bed your temperature should be around 98 degrees; at midmorning after you've had breakfast and been up and around for a while, it should be normal—98.6 degrees. This temperature should be maintained until early evening when it begins to drop to around 98 degrees. Any temperature reading below these numbers indicates an underactive thyroid. When you're on thyroid medication and your temperature normalizes without causing an increase in the heart rate or pulse, you know you're taking enough medication to maintain normal thyroid function.

You can get an idea of whether foods depress your thyroid function by taking your temperature a half hour after eating a single food and then one hour after that. (This shouldn't be confused with the pulse test.) A below-normal temperature after eating a single food item is a pretty good indication of a food allergy. Drinking three cups of tea caused my temperature to fall by about one degree; after six cups of tea it dropped an additional degree. When I drink only one cup of tea, my 98.5 temperature remains steady.

The basal thermometer test may be the best overall test for hypothyroidism, because it measures what is most critical—the amount of energy generated inside the cell. However, there are other factors responsible for slow thyroid activity that should be measured. Most medical doctors rely solely on the TSH test to measure thyroid function. But you should take the following thyroid tests because each one tests something different: free T4, free T3, reverse T3, total T4, and total T3, as well as the thyroglobulin antibodies (TGA) test.

A thyroid test doctors rarely give is the reverse T3, probably because elevated reverse T3 is not a common cause of hypothyroidism. While regular T3 tells the energy-producing mitochondria in the cells how much energy to produce, reverse T3 blocks the regular T3 from entering the cells, with the result that energy production decreases.

The reverse T3 blocks energy production when there is too little intake of food. Thus in times of famine when there is not enough glucose or fat in the body, reverse T3 levels rise in order to lower energy production so that body fat and glucose are conserved.

When food becomes plentiful, reverse T3 blood levels drop far below that of regular T3, because with the intake of enough food there is no need to conserve body fuel. If despite the fact that you are eating enough, and your regular T3 level is normal, you still have the symptoms of an underactive thyroid, it may be because your reverse T3 levels are too high.[2]

Why do a few individuals, although having plenty to eat, nevertheless have high levels of reverse T3? Dr. Richard Cordaro, a chiropractor and nutritionist in New York City, has found that nearly all individuals with excessive levels of reverse T3 suffer from heavy metal accumulation. Cordaro says that by removing the cadmium, mercury, lead, and other heavy metals from the body, reverse T3 levels are lowered and symptoms of hypothyroidism lessen or disappear altogether.[3]

A dependable method for detecting heavy metal levels in the blood is the chelation test. Amino acids are injected into the blood where they bond with heavy metal molecules and are eliminated through the urine. After an injection, the urine is monitored for heavy metals over the next six hours.

You can't assume, because all the tests you take point to low thyroid function, that the trouble originates with the thyroid. It's possible that the parathyroid, the gland that regulates blood calcium levels, is responsible. Dr. Cordaro says that if a patient has a problem with the parathyroid, it's a sign that thyroid function is also not normal, and the reverse is equally true.[4] So, whether a patient comes to him with a thyroid or a parathyroid problem, Cordaro treats both glands. (See "Suggestions for the Maintenance of Normal Thyroid Function" at the end of the chapter for the supplements he recommends.)

An underactive thyroid can also be due to a deficiency of progesterone. Have your progesterone levels tested; if they are too low, ask your doctor to prescribe a natural progesterone cream or progesterone supplements (see the suggestions in Chapter 16).

Elevated Blood Pressure Can Indicate a Low-Functioning Thyroid

If you're fifty or older, you can get a pretty good idea of how well your thyroid is functioning by taking your blood pressure. In my experience, when blood pressure is elevated, body temperature tends to be below normal, indicating that toxic debris from inappropriate food and heavy metals have raised the blood pressure by slowing down thyroid function. Monitoring your body temperature and your blood pressure to find out what foods are incompatible with your metabolism and then avoiding them is the most effective way to maintain normal thyroid function and good overall health. It's hard to imagine that anyone age fifty or older who has both normal thyroid function and normal blood pressure could be suffering from any sort of degenerative illness. In most older people, acidic waste from bad diet has already lowered thyroid function and raised blood pressure. Various studies indicate that anywhere from 50 to 90 percent of the population has a thyroid insufficiency.[5] If these figures were broken down by age, I'm sure it would show that nearly 100 percent of those over the age of fifty have an underactive thyroid—and that those who don't have a hyperactive thyroid! Individuals in their twenties, thirties, and sometimes even in their forties can eat junk food and still have normal thyroid function because they have enough enzymes to neutralize excessive levels of acid waste which interfere with thyroid function. But by late middle age some enzyme-producing glands have worn out from overwork.

Reduce Acidic Waste to Revive Thyroid Function

Allergy-causing foods, inappropriate diet, and heavy metal accumulation create acidic waste. Circulating in the blood, this waste can lodge in the capillaries near the thyroid, blocking the flow of tyrosine (an amino acid) and iodine, the raw materials that go into the thyroid's production of thyroxin (T4). Acidic wastes can also clog the liver. This further reduces energy production, since the liver is responsible for converting T4 to the active T3.

Toxic waste in the blood also throws hormone levels out of balance. By elevating estrogen, it lowers progesterone, the hormone that is "thyroid friendly." Detoxification of the liver with vitamins E and C, and avoidance of junk food and foods your digestive system can't handle, heals the liver and restores its ability to convert T4 into its active form (T3).

Foods That Suppress Thyroid Function

There are also substances in certain foods that suppress thyroid function. These foods should be avoided if you have an underactive thyroid: beans (all beans except string beans); peanuts; polyunsaturated oils; undercooked broccoli, cauliflower, and cabbage; muscle meat; and beta-carotene. Goiter (enlarged thyroid) ceased to be a major health problem when iodine was added to salt, but more recently, with the use of iodide as an emulsifier in bread dough, yogurt, and pudding to make a smooth consistency, the public is getting an overload of iodine. This can interfere with the thyroid's production of thyroxin to the same extent as too little iodine and is probably one of the causes of the current epidemic of hypothyroidism. Foods that promote thyroid function are animal hearts, butter, vitamin A instead of beta-carotene, skin for its gelatin content (unless you are sensitive to MSG [monosodium glutamate]), and eggs.[6]

Avoid Processed Foods and Water Pollutants

As discussed earlier, thyroid function is also inhibited by the heavy metal residues found in processed foods and in food additives. Estrogen, a stress hormone, can increase the heavy metal levels in our bodies because it stimulates the absorption of iron. Excess iron depletes oxygen needed for respiration (energy production). Avoiding processed foods that are contaminated with heavy metals improves thyroid function and lowers excess estrogen levels. This in turn prevents surplus iron from being stored in the body, which in older people becomes a problem, as an aging body absorbs heavy metals more readily than a young one.

Low thyroxin levels in the blood, which inhibit thyroid function, are also caused by water pollutants. Sir Robert McCarrison, a British physician who spent a lifetime traveling to remote areas of the world looking for the cause of goiter, found one answer on the side of a mountain in Kashmir, India. Nine villages, built one above the other, shared the same water supply that flowed in a channel down the mountain. This water served every purpose: drinking and cooking, irrigation of crops, bathing, washing utensils and clothes, as a latrine, and as a basin for catching manure-saturated runoff water from cultivated fields. While the water was relatively clean at the top of the mountain, as it flowed downward it gradually filled with organic pollutants so that the lower a village was situated the more polluted the water and the greater the incidence of goiters. It would be hard to find a cause of goiter among the people in these nine villages other than the amount of pollution in their water supply, since the incidence of goiter in each village correlated directly with the degree of pollution in the water they used.

In the United States there isn't a problem with organic water pollutants, since chlorine, a poisonous gas added to the water supply, kills off the bacteria that live off organic waste. There is no mineral, however, that neutralizes the toxic chemicals that have infiltrated the groundwater tables. Examples of water contamination by chemical wastes are resorcinol and dihydroxol, by-products of coal-mining operations in Kentucky. These have been discovered in the water supplies in towns in the Appalachian Mountains, where there is a high incidence of goiter, especially among children. Fluoridated water is also an inhibitor of thyroid function. Because the thyroid absorbs waterborne pollutants so easily, it's difficult to maintain normal thyroid function unless water used for drinking and cooking has been distilled or comes from underground springs that are tested regularly.

There isn't a mental or physical health problem in existence that can't be caused by an underactive thyroid—and therefore not one that can't be improved by normalizing thyroid function. The prime factor in maintaining a normal thyroid is the original source of energy that maintains every living thing on earth: direct sunlight, which is converted into chemical energy (ATP). ATP is imbedded in the glucose molecules of the food we eat. It provides the raw material for cellular respiration. We obtain a supply of chemical energy when we eat, say, a banana. After it is digested, some of the glucose molecules in the banana are carried by the bloodstream to the mitochondria in the cells, where they are split up to release their energy. This chemical energy is converted to heat energy. But for this respiratory process to take place, red light, the longest light wave of the sun, must be present. Gaining entry into the body through the eyes and skin, the red spectrum rays of sunlight are carried by the blood to the pineal gland. The pigment in the pineal absorbs it, just as light is absorbed into the chlorophyll pigment in the chloroplasts in leaves for the production of glucose.

There are still relatively unpolluted areas in the mountains and national parks in the United States where you can expose your body to a few weeks of good quality sunlight a year—the most important factor in the body's ability to generate energy.

SUGGESTIONS FOR THE MAINTENANCE OF NORMAL THYROID FUNCTION*

➤ If tests indicate you have low thyroid function, have your parathyroid and progesterone tested (both men and women). If they are underactive, they may be responsible for your sluggish thyroid function.

➤ If your temperature is subnormal, check for food allergies (see Chapter 2) before you start taking thyroid supplements.

➤ If you can't normalize your thyroid function with nutritional supplements (outlined here) take a medication that contains T3 as well as T4, such as CynoPlus. Medications that contain only T4 are dangerous. If the liver is sluggish and can't convert all the T4 into the active T3, the excess T4 suppresses thyroid function. So as not to overload the liver with T4, break the thyroid tablet into two pieces, and take one half in the morning and the other half at night.

➤ Dr. Cordaro recommends for both hypothyroid and hyperthyroid problems a glandular called Thytrophin (made by Standard Process) as well as the herb bladderwrack for hypothyroid and bugleweed for hyperthyroid. He always includes in his treatment of the thyroid gland a Standard Process product called Calma Plus for the parathyroid (it's a type of calcium specifically designed for this gland). (After taking glandulars for a while, drug medication is sometimes no longer necessary.)

➤ Get exposure to sunlight preferably daily when the sun is at an angle, so as to reduce exposure to ultraviolet light. To maximize your exposure to sunlight, try panning (take off glasses, close your eyes, raise your head toward the sun, and move your head slowly from side to side).

➤ Taking 400 to 800 units a day of vitamin E helps normalize thyroid function whether you have an underactive or overactive thyroid.

➤ Taking 25,000 units a day of vitamin A converts cholesterol to progesterone, the thyroid-friendly hormone.

➤ A mineral complex, preferably in liquid form, helps in the conversion of tyrosine, an amino acid, to thyroxin and also the conversion of T4 to T3 in the liver.

➤ Orange and grapefruit juices are good sources of glucose and minerals to ensure normal respiration. The minerals such as magnesium, potassium, and sodium in these citrus juices are present in the right balance, and the sugar in the juice provides the fuel needed by the respiratory organelles for the manufacture of the form of energy the body uses for organ function.

➤ Vitamin B complex and vitamin C help eliminate side effects of thyroid drug medication in individuals with hardening of the arteries.

➤ Two teaspoons a day of coconut oil, an additional source of fuel, counteracts the toxic effects of polyunsaturated oils on the thyroid gland.

➤ Raw eggs promote thyroid and progesterone function and protect the fat in the body from degenerating. Use only eggs laid by hens fed organically grown grain.

➤ Progesterone for women and pregnenolone for men is helpful for those who have an underactive thyroid. Natural progesterone cream should be applied locally wherever the blood vessels are close to the skin, for example, on the neck or wrist. The molecular structure of natural progesterone is the same as that of progesterone produced by the human body. The synthetic hormone progestin has a different structure. Progestin, along with estrogen derived from mares'

continued

urine, in the hormone replacement therapy preparation has been implicated in female reproductive cancer. (See Resources.)

➤ Pregnenolone normalizes a hyperactive thyroid, whose symptoms are bulging eyes and Graves disease. Take 1 to 5 mg daily of natural pregnenolone. Go off it periodically for one week.

---

* Take as many of these nutrients as possible in the form of whole-food complexes. For dosage, follow the directions on the label.

CHAPTER 6

CARDIOVASCULAR DISEASE

S am, my colleague at City College, born and raised on the African coast of Ghana, had a father who died at the age of 103 in full possession of his mental faculties. Sam believed he had inherited his father's longevity genes, since in looks and mind-set he was his carbon copy. His father, however, unlike Sam, had eaten healthy foods all his life. His dietary staple was fish that he ate right after he had caught and cleaned it, yams and cassava he dug up from the earth and threw into the fire minutes before he devoured them, and coconut milk he drank straight from the shell as soon as he got up in the morning. He sprinkled his food with what is considered the best salt in the world—mineral rich, reddish colored, and sweet tasting, it is raked up from the shoreline of the Ghana coast. Sam, on the other hand, having immigrated to the United States as a young man, had eaten processed foods most of his life. Now at age 86 his chances of living to be as old as his father were slim, since he was suffering from hardening of the arteries, a disease unknown among Ghanans—despite their high intake of salt.

I recommended to Sam that he change his diet instead of having an angioplasty, but he followed his doctors' advice and went ahead with the operation. In this procedure, a balloon is threaded through the arteries to the heart and expanded. After clearing away the plaque blocking the arteries, the surgeon implants a stent to keep the artery open, thus assuring the maximum flow of blood. The operation appeared at first to be a success. With his arteries cleared, Sam's chest pains went away and the increased flow of blood through the widened arteries now carried a sufficient supply of oxygen to the cells for the production of energy. Once again full of vigor, Sam no longer swayed and tottered when he walked, and his voice lost the gravelly sound typical of people with advanced heart disease.

Sam's return to health, however, was short-lived. The first symptom indicating his cardiovascular problems had returned was the slowing of his heartbeat. This is typically caused by an increase in estrogen (a sign that his testosterone levels had become deficient). Too much estrogen in the blood causes the veins carrying blood back to the heat to expand too much. This delays the return of the blood to the heart with the result that the heartbeat slows its pace. Within six months the inside walls of his arteries were once again encrusted with calcified plaque.

Acidic Waste and Cardiovascular Problems

What caused Sam's arteries to harden after they had been cleared of cholesterol, calcium, and various other kinds of debris? A question more to the point is, *why did they harden in the first place?* As usual, scientific researchers have looked in the wrong direction. Ignoring the true cause of the calcified plaques lining the arteries—injuries inflicted on the arteries by sharp crystals of acidic waste—they have come up with a culprit called cytomegalovirus that invades the body and implants itself inside the walls of the arteries.

Several studies support the connection between the presence of this virus and the regrowth of plaque. In one study of seventy-five patients who had had an angioplasty, fatty plaque recurred in 75 percent of those patients who were infected with the cytomegalovirus, while only 8 percent who were not infected had a recurrence of plaque. Another study shows that patients with no symptoms of heart disease who were taking tetracycline were 30 percent less likely than those who were not taking antibiotics to have a heart attack.[1]

Virus and Bacteria from Acidic Waste Cause Arterial Hardening

This would seem to be solid evidence that the cytomegalovirus is the cause of artery hardening. The fact is, however, that the presence in the arteries of this virus is explained by the acidic waste (from undigested food debris) circulating in the blood. Viruses and bacteria thrive and multiply on acidic waste. In this regard it is instructive to remember the bitter conclusion that the famous German pathologist Rudolf Virchow (1821–1902) came to after spending a lifetime doing research based on the belief that germs were the cause of disease: "If I could live my life over again I would devote it to proving that germs seek their natural habitat—diseased tissue. For example, mosquitoes seek the stagnant water but do not cause the pool to become stagnant."[2]

Studies demonstrate that in the short term, antibiotics, vaccines, and strong anti-inflammatory drugs eliminate megalovirus infections, preventing the regrowth of plaque after an angioplasty. But no studies have been made on the long-term effectiveness of these treatments. It seems unlikely that the health of the arteries can be maintained indefinitely even with the use of antibiotics to kill off the cytomegalovirus, when the condition that caused the original inflammation is not addressed—the acid waste circulating in the arterial blood that damages the arteries and provides nourishment for the cytomegalovirus.[3]

In nature, bacteria and viruses live off the acidic tissue of dead organisms—they are nature's primary decomposers. The acid waste

THE CONSEQUENCES OF HIGH BLOOD PRESSURE

High blood pressure occurs when the walls of the blood vessels become constricted and cause a rise in the pressure exerted by the blood against the blood vessel walls. If the blood vessels are healthy (that is, if they are not inflamed or hardened), they can take this added pressure without being injured or endangering the heart. If there is some hardening in the arteries, however, constricted blood vessels can cause a heart attack or stroke because increased pressure on arteries and veins encrusted with calcified plaques can force a calcified plaque loose. This triggers the formation of a blood clot. Taking vitamin E—preferably in a whole-food complex—can prevent blood clots, as vitamin E is a natural blood thinner.

from undigested food circulating in the blood provides germs in the blood with the same kind of acidic brew that the dead bodies of wild animals and plants provide the bacteria in nature.

Acidic waste particles make scratches and tears on the inside walls of the blood vessels. The injured cells die off and turn into acidic waste, adding to its accumulation in the blood. The larger the quantities of acidic waste the greater the food supply for germs; they multiply correspondingly. This forces the immune system to defend the walls of the arteries by triggering the growth of tumors to encapsulate germ colonies, causing further damage to the arterial walls.

The immune system also patches the injuries in the lining of the vessels with calcified plaques to prevent life-threatening leaks, and it reacts to arterial degeneration the same way it does to bodily injury from accidents—by triggering the flow of blood to the area that inflames the walls of the arteries. These measures prevent imminent death but set up the conditions for a heart attack. All that has to occur is for a blood clot to form, blocking the flow of blood to the heart. This can occur when a calcified plaque on the vessel wall breaks loose.

The most common symptoms of a heart attack are nausea, a feeling of suffocation, dizziness and fainting episodes, tightness in the chest, or pain in the region of the heart or left shoulder accompanied by feelings of anxiety. If, however, a pain in the chest occurs at the same time as the hands and feet become cold and breath becomes short, it is usually a sign of indigestion.

The Cholesterol Issue

Why was the role of "bad guy" in coronary heart disease assigned to cholesterol—that waxy, gray-yellow substance in our bodies that is vital to the growth of tissue, development of the brain, and manufacture of hormones? The answer lies in the mind-set of the medical establishment, which holds that when a medical problem arises, a "bad guy" is responsible: a virus, bacteria, or some substance researchers label harmful, which the body itself manufactures—such as cholesterol.

Medical researchers have ignored studies conducted by Rudolf Virchow in the nineteenth century. He discovered that degeneration of the blood vessels started before cholesterol plaques appeared in the lesions.

The late Dr. G. E. Barnes reaffirmed Virchow's conclusions. He examined fifty thousand autopsies of people who died in Europe during World War II when saturated fats like meat and butter were scarce. These autopsies showed advanced hardening of the arteries in spite of the low-cholesterol diet in individuals who had died too young to have heart attacks. Legions of statistics show similar results, among them the fourteen-year Framingham, Massachusetts, study, which found that one-half of the individuals in the study who died of heart attacks had normal cholesterol levels.[4] This indicates that there is no definitive link between moderately high cholesterol and cardiovascular disease.

Inflammation and Heart Disease

Another condition related to heart disease is inflammation of the inside walls of the veins and arteries. This connection, unlike the cholesterol connection, has been established in many studies. One such study, published in the November 2002 issue of the *New England Journal of Medicine*, found that men whose arteries have been inflamed for several years are three times more likely to have heart attacks and two times more likely to have strokes as individuals whose arteries are not inflamed.[5] Researchers point to a body chemical called C-reactive protein (CRP) as the inflammatory agent, and medications are now prescribed that lower blood CRP levels.

Studies that came out in 2008 found that people with high CRP levels (although low in LDL cholesterol) who took statins (drugs that inhibit the synthesis of cholesterol) had fewer heart attacks. As a result of these findings, it was taken for granted that elevated CRP was a cause of heart attacks. The puzzling results of a new study on the inflammatory effects of CRP muddy the issue. Conducted by *JAMA* in 2009 on more than one hundred thousand subjects,[6] the study revealed that different people produce different amounts of CRP, yet those who make more CRP don't have more heart attacks than those who make less of it. For such people, taking drug medications to lower their CRP levels is not necessary and may even be dangerous.

The fact is that those whose elevated CRP levels are the result of inflamed arteries are far more likely than people with genetically elevated CRP levels to have heart attacks. Thus, a high level of CRP doesn't necessarily correlate with a high level of inflammation. Only when the arteries are inflamed should an elevated CRP be taken seriously.

Heart Disease and Hormonal Imbalance

There is a relationship between heart disease and hormonal imbalance that is worth noting. Excessive acid waste in the blood from anxiety or poor diet triggers the rise of the stress-promoting hormones estrogen and cortisol. At unacceptably high levels, these hormones trigger heart

---

DIRK MAKES A COMPLETE RECOVERY FROM A HEART ATTACK

Dirk Collier was forty-eight years old and president and CEO of a Fortune 500 financial services company when he had a heart attack. He had just finished playing a tennis match when he felt a sharp pain around his heart and numbness in his left arm. His tennis partner called an ambulance, which delivered him to the nearest hospital. Tests confirmed that Dirk had had a coronary occlusion. Dirk couldn't believe that he was sitting in bed with a damaged heart, pain in his chest, and out of breath, when, for the past ten years he had jogged every day and taken a multiple vitamin and mineral complex, a B complex, and vitamin C. There was one vitamin he had overlooked, however, and that was vitamin E. The 50 units of E in his multivitamin was not enough to prevent his blood from clotting if he lacked the antithrombin (anticlotting) factor. Dirk began taking 800 units of a vitamin E supplement that included all the tocopherols.

After six weeks he had not regained his energy, so he doubled the dosage to 1,600 units. A month later Dirk felt a return of his strength and noticed the pain in his chest had vanished. Now, twenty-seven years later, in retirement in Scottsdale, Arizona, he feels well enough to play tennis three times a week. He continues to take vitamin E—in the form of a whole-food vitamin E supplement called Cataplex E2—along with the other supplements he had taken before his heart attack.

disease. Excess estrogen does so by destroying oxygen, which inflames the arteries and veins. Estrogen has also been found to expand the walls of the veins carrying blood back to the heart, postponing the return of the blood to the heart and causing the heartbeat to slow.[7]

Elevated cortisol and estrogen levels due to stress can also provoke heart attacks by acidifying the blood. Life-promoting hormones like pregnenolone (for men) and progesterone (for women) can lower estrogen and cortisol levels. Heart patients need to take the natural form of progesterone or pregnenolone to reduce these stress-promoting hormones. Once the stress-promoting hormones are lowered, the acidic waste, whose injuries to the arterial walls was what caused the calcified plaques to form in the first place, is reduced and the arterial walls begin to heal. Finally the calcified plaques dissolve and are eliminated.

Natural progesterone and other natural life-promoting hormones have been widely used in Europe for the past fifty years. Numerous studies conducted in Europe show these hormones to have no undesirable side effects. They improve circulation, do away with calcified plaques in the arteries, and heal inflamed tissue. An additional advantage to using progesterone is that it is converted as needed to other hormones.

Neutralize Acidic Waste for Cardiovascular Health

How did vitamin E heal Dirk's cardiovascular system? Its anticlotting factor prevented the formation of blood clots, and its oxygenation of the blood neutralized the acidic waste that provides food for bacteria and injures the lining of the vessels and heart. Without the presence of these toxic acid particles, the self-healing powers of the circulating system went into effect.

Individuals who suffer from hypoxia (oxygen deficiency) are more vulnerable to heart disease. But it is not easy to recognize hypoxia. I had it. One of my symptoms was an inability to stand still for longer than five minutes without feeling faint. I began taking vitamin E, and two months later I was able to stand for any length of time without feeling light-headed. The vitamin E had overcome the oxygen deficiency in my brain.

The B vitamins are also important in the prevention of cardiovascular disease. Their beneficial effects, although discovered more than thirty years ago, have only recently been brought to light. Dr. Kilmer McCully of Harvard University discovered that deficiencies in vitamins B_6, B_{12}, and folic acid gave rise to abnormally high levels of an amino acid called homocysteine. This turned out to be a major factor in heart disease. The leftover homocysteine turns into acidic waste because there are not enough B vitamins to dispose of it. Many studies confirm the importance of the B vitamins in promoting a healthy heart. For example, one study found that people who took B-vitamin supplements had half the heart disease rate of those who didn't.[8] These studies indicate that healthy people should take B vitamins as a heart attack and stroke preventative.

Other nutrients essential to heart health include magnesium (an anticoagulant), vitamin C, copper, and hawthorn berry liquid extract. Hawthorn berries' wide-ranging healing powers are due in great part to the fact that its beneficial effects begin as soon as it is swallowed and enters the digestive tract. The berries' abundant food-digesting enzymes step up the speed at which food in the stomach is broken down, so there is little undigested food left to acidify. Hawthorn berries also contain an alkaline factor that binds with acidic particles and neutralizes them. When a minimum of acidic waste is formed in the digestive tract, the arteries, veins, and kidneys have a chance to heal, and the fatty plaque "bandages," no longer needed, are dissolved and carried away by the blood.

The health of the heart and the arteries also depends on a balance between fats from fish and green, leafy vegetables and those from meat and butter. A recent study of people in Japan and the Mediterranean countries showed that those whose diet is rich in omega-3 fatty acids from eating green, leafy vegetables and fish have a lower incidence of heart disease than those who are big meat eaters.[9] But what must be considered here is that the people in these countries are by virtue of their grain-eating metabolisms far more likely to be healthier when they conform to their indigenous grain and fish diet—just as those living in northern Europe are more likely to have healthy hearts if they conform to their meat-eating diet.

SUGGESTIONS FOR CARDIOVASCULAR HEALTH*

➤ **Progesterone.** Use a natural form of progesterone in the form of a cream. Follow the directions on the label.

➤ **Pregnenolone.** This hormone is especially effective in men. Don't take too much pregnenolone. It can cause headaches, irritability, and lack of energy. Taking 1 or 2 mg daily with periodic time-outs of one week is enough for most people.

➤ **Red rice yeast** (600 to 1,200 mg daily) **with Ubiquinol** (activated form of CoQ-10; 150 to 300 mg daily). This is the best protocol for lowering cholesterol. Ubiquinol, which increases energy production in the heart, prevents liver damage from the red rice yeast. (Statins also cause liver damage, but doctors don't have a remedy.) If your cholesterol reading is over 300, take the maximum dose of both supplements. If you are switching from a statin to red rice yeast, consult an alternative health-care practitioner.

➤ **Niacin** (3 to 5 g/day). Niacin not only lowers cholesterol but also removes arterial plaque.

➤ **Cataplex E2.** A whole food vitamin E complex. Follow the directions on the bottle. After taking regular vitamin E until heart symptoms are eliminated, add Cataplex E2 to your nutritional supplement regimen.

➤ **Vitamin C** (500 units/day).

➤ **Vitamin A** (20,000 units/day). Vitamin A promotes synthesis of progesterone and pregnenolone.

➤ **Vitamin E.** If you've had a heart attack, begin taking 800 units a day. Increase the dose by 200 units every six weeks until your symptoms disappear. Don't take more than 1,600 units. For heart disease prevention, women should take 400 units daily, men 800 units, and children no more than 100 units.

➤ **Vitamin B complex.** Find a complex that contains at least 50 mg of B_1, B_2, B_3, and B_6. Your daily intake of folic acid should be 1,000 mcg/day. For prevention, take 800 mcg/day of folic acid,

continued

along with 500 mcg/day of B_{12} (take the sublingual tablet) and 100 mg/day of B_6.

➤ **Hawthorn berry extract.** Begin with 20 drops and work up to 50 drops three times a day. Even if you don't have heart disease, when you reach the age of fifty, take 20 drops twice a day to prevent decomposition of the heart. Hawthorn berry extract lowers blood pressure by dilating the peripheral blood vessels.

➤ **Devil's claw.** This herb is the most effective supplement for lowering blood pressure.

➤ **Taurine** (2 to 4 g/day). This amino acid is used extensively in Japan to treat congestive heart failure and heart arrhythmias (irregularities).

➤ **Liquid mineral complex.** Look for one that includes at least 400 mg of calcium, potassium, and magnesium and 200 mcg selenium. Follow the directions on the bottle.

➤ **Thyroid supplement** (preferably Thytrophin, a glandular made by Standard Process). It speeds up the efficiency with which waste products are eliminated from the body by accelerating the metabolism.

➤ **CoQ-10.** This coenzyme is involved in the production and transportation of energy in the heart. There is more CoQ-10 in the heart than in any other organ. The heart patient should take 150 mg/day of Ubiquinol, the activated form of CoQ-10. For maintenance of the cardiovascular system, take 30 mg/day.

➤ **Carpain.** This is an enzyme found in papaya, which is good for the heart.

➤ **Hot water with lemon juice.** Drink this first thing in the morning. It removes plaques from arterial walls, detoxifies the liver, and stimulates the production of food-digesting enzymes.

➤ **Cooked asparagus and raw or cooked celery.** The arsenic in these vegetables, which is in phosphate form and therefore not dangerous, aids in the regeneration of heart tissue.

➤ **Watermelon.** This fruit has 60 percent more lycopene than tomatoes. It strengthens the heart as well as the prostate.

➤ **Cetyl myristate.** Six tablets daily of this fatty acid lowers high blood pressure caused by hardening of the arteries. (See Resources.)

➤ **Pycnogenol** (50 mg twice a day). Extracted from pine bark, it's the most easily assimilated bioflavonoid. It reduces inflammation and strengthens the inner lining of blood vessels, so it's also effective for varicose veins. Pycnogenol helps dissolve blood clots in phlebitis.

➤ **Wobenzyme.** Take two capsules with each meal. It is an effective anti-inflammatory enzyme and also aids in digestion.

➤ **L-carnitine** (1,500 to 3,000 units/day). L-carnitine decreases cholesterol and triglycerides and aids in the transport of fatty acid used by the heart to manufacture energy.

*Take as many as possible of these nutrients in the form of whole-food complexes. Follow the directions on the bottle for dosage.

CHAPTER 7

KIDNEY DISEASE

Everyone who has ever watched boxing knows there is one part of the body it is against the rules to punch—the lower back where the kidneys are located. The kidneys are vulnerable because in the center of each kidney are filters called nephrons that are very fragile. They filter the blood, thus keeping the acid-alkaline pH of the blood balanced and removing toxins that could cause toxemia (blood poisoning). The networks of blood vessels that encircle each nephron—they are microscopic and number in the millions—filter out water, urea, glucose, minerals, and enzymes from the blood. Most of these compounds are reabsorbed into the main bloodstream. What's left behind—excess water, salt, urea, and uric acid—is excreted as urine.

If water, salt, urea, and a small amount of uric acid were all that the kidneys had to remove from the blood, kidney failure would be unknown. However, to prevent death from toxemia, which is to say, excessive levels of acid, the kidneys filter out the kind of highly toxic acidic waste they weren't designed to handle.

The Kidney's Role in Filtering Acidic Wastes

There are many different kinds of acids coursing through the blood that are left to the kidneys to dispose of. There is the mercury, lead, iron, cadmium, and aluminum from immunization shots. (The polio vaccine contains twenty-eight compounds foreign to the body, including formaldehyde, an embalming fluid.) The vaccine immunization program given to children, starting at birth, is estimated to have caused millions of cases of kidney degeneration in the young.[1] A major source of acidic waste the kidneys have to filter out of the blood is the end-products of protein digestion. For example, the liver neutralizes serum protein by converting it into salts. When it is unable to do so, the kidneys have to filter out this strong acid "as is." The kidneys are also burdened at times with the removal of acetic, lactic, and sulfuric acid, the by-products of protein that the overworked liver hasn't had the time or sufficient energy to neutralize. And when insulin levels are too low to normalize high blood sugar levels, the kidneys have to filter out the excess sugar from the blood as well.

As these sharp acidic particles stream through the capillaries in the nephrons, they act like harsh cleaning solvents, scraping and scratching the inside walls of these fragile micro blood vessels. And just as injured arteries are patched up with calcium-encrusted fatty plaques, so the damaged walls of these capillaries in the kidneys get filled in with microscopic particles of calcium and fat. While it usually takes decades before arteries become hardened, the tiny capillaries in the kidneys are stopped up in much less time.

As nephrons are knocked out, the remaining filters need more plasma (fluid) in the blood to strain out the filtrate (the solid part of the blood) if they are to do so without sustaining injury. The hormones comply by increasing the volume of the blood. The downside is that with the increase in blood volume, blood pressure rises. Doctors react by pre-scribing a diuretic, which lowers the blood pressure by removing some of the liquid plasma from the blood. Because this narrows the ratio between the plasma (fluid) and solid components in the blood, the nephrons are once again more likely to be damaged as they filter out solid particles from the blood plasma. The nephrons are injured in another way as well. Once the acids cause the arteries in the general circulatory system to harden so they can no longer absorb the pressure of the circulating blood, the kidneys have to bear the impact.

It is thought that the nephron filters in the kidneys, unlike the liver and even the lungs, have no regenerative power. Contradicting this belief is the result of my recommendations of vitamin E to patients afflicted with polycystic kidneys, end-stage lupus, and kidney failure.

In all three cases, vitamin E brought back much of the nephrons' filtering function.

Kidneys and Water Consumption

One of the kidneys' tasks is to regulate the concentration of salts in the body. When the kidneys' management of salt metabolism is normal, each atom of sodium picks up twenty-one molecules of water, which is excreted from the body as urine. The fact that urine enters the bladder from the kidneys drop by drop gives an indication of how slowly the kidneys filter water and waste products out of the blood. When water is gulped down so fast that it pours into the digestive tract like water from a faucet turned on full, it stretches the walls of the capillaries in the nephrons to the breaking point. The best way to synchronize drinking water with the rate at which the kidneys process it is to sip it slowly. You can satisfy a great part of your water requirements by eating the raw vegetables and fruit that have the highest percentage of water, such as tomatoes, cucumbers, lettuce, and oranges. The much slower process of eating as opposed to drinking ensures that the amount of water ingested at any given time won't be more than the kidneys can filter out of the blood in the same amount of time.

MALCOLM: ONE STEP AWAY FROM DIALYSIS

Malcolm had been on diuretics to lower his high blood pressure for more than twenty years. From the time I made his acquaintance, five years ago, he looked haggard with huge bags under his eyes, the latter often a sign of poor kidney function. He came up to me recently at a meeting and told me he had kidney failure. He asked if I had any suggestions. His was the classic case of kidney failure caused by the high blood pressure medication he had been taking for so long. On questioning him further he told me that 30 percent of his nephrons (filters) were still working but

continued

that his doctor predicted that in a few months they would wear out like the others had. At that point he would have to go on dialysis.

I suggested that for the next three months he tax his kidneys as little as possible. I prescribed nothing but juices made from organic vegetables, starting out with bland vegetables such as zucchinis and lettuce, a week later adding celery and shortly after one medium-sized organic potato for the protein and carbohydrates he needed to sustain him for the three months he was on a liquid diet. Because he was a borderline diabetic, he couldn't have carrot juice. Vegetables with a bitter taste are considered by traditional cultures to be effective in lowering blood sugar. Malcolm juiced bitter melon that he bought at a market in Chinatown. To satisfy the body's fat and oil requirements he took two pats of organic butter along with some organic olive oil, once a day the first week and twice a day thereafter. Because I've had such success in bringing failed kidneys back to life with 1,600 units of vitamin E a day, I suggested that Malcolm begin taking this two weeks after he started juicing. He also began to take devil's claw, an herb that reduces blood pressure, at the same time. As the herb took effect, his doctor gradually took him off diarvan, his blood pressure medication. This was two years ago, and Malcolm's remaining nephrons are still functioning.

Preventing the Recurrence of Kidney Stones

The effect of a heavy meat diet on the formation of kidney stones is made clear in an experiment described in an article in the *Journal of Urology*.[2] Because of increasing contact with the West since World War II, the Japanese have been eating more meat and fewer vegetables. To find out whether this change in diet was responsible for tripling the rate of kidney stones among the Japanese, researchers at Kinki University in Osaka conducted a study. They divided 370 men into two groups and put each on a different diet. One group was on a low-meat, high-vegetable diet, and the other simply increased their intake of fluids. It turned out that the men on a diet of mostly vegetables and little meat were 40 to 60 percent less likely to have a recurrence of kidney stones than the group with increased fluids only.

The problem with large quantities of meat in the diet is that urea, the by-product of protein breakdown, causes too much urine to be excreted. This has the effect of throwing out the baby with the bath-water, because alkaline-forming mineral molecules are excreted along with the urea when urine output is excessive. Without enough alkalinizing minerals to neutralize acid waste in the blood, the urine becomes highly acidic. The greater number of acidic particles in the urine the more likely they are to stick together. When enough of these particles adhere to each other, they form a stone.

Kidney stones are usually composed of calcium and oxalic acid. What most people with kidney stones don't know is that oxalic acid, like calcium, performs a vital function. Ninety-eight percent of the oxalic acid in the body is produced internally and is used for moving food through the digestive tract by peristalsis (the contraction and relaxation of muscles). Oxalic acid also aids in the absorption of calcium into the cells.

Leftover oxalic acid, along with excess calcium, is removed from the blood by the kidneys and passes into the urine. Calcium oxalate permeates the urine generally, but only in those people whose urine is over-loaded with acid waste does it form stones.

It would seem that the way to prevent kidney stones would be to alkalinize the urine. But urologists, unaware apparently that the pH factor in the urine determines whether or not stones are formed, recommend reducing the levels of calcium and oxalic acid in the diet. Kidney stone patients are instructed not to eat any green vegetables, especially broccoli, which is high in calcium, and spinach, beet greens, and chard because of their high oxalic acid content. By doing so, doctors are depriving their patients of valuable nutrients, one of which, calcium, actually helps prevent kidney stones by alkalinizing the urine.

It's probably a good idea for anyone who has a tendency to form stones to go easy on cooked spinach, beet greens, and rhubarb, the only foods that are extremely high in oxalates (although oxalates from these foods constitute only 2 percent of the oxalates in the body, hardly enough to be considered responsible for creating stones). These greens, however, can be eaten in generous amounts if they are raw.

SUGGESTIONS FOR KIDNEY STONES AND NEPHRITIS*

➤ **Magnesium oxide and vitamin B$_6$.** A 1999 study showed that individuals with recurrent kidney stones on 300 mg/day of magnesium oxide and 10 mg/day of vitamin B$_6$ dropped their recurrence rate from 1.3 to 0.1 kidney stones per year.[3]

➤ **Vitamin E** (800 to 1,600 units/day). Vitamin E reduces inflammation through its oxygenating effect.

➤ **Vitamin A.** Start out with 50,000 units/day for three months; 25,000 units/day thereafter.

➤ **Cranberry juice.** Drink eight ounces three times daily.

➤ **Vitamin C** (1,000 mg/day).

➤ **Raw asparagus juice.** Drink eight ounces twice daily.

➤ **Choline** (250 mg/day).

➤ **Low consumption of meat.** Eat no more than seven ounces daily.

➤ **Vegetables—raw, whole, and juiced.** Vegetables should be the major part of the diet until the kidney stones are dissolved and/or the inflammation is gone.

➤ **Hot water with the juice of one lemon.** Drink one glass every day in the morning upon waking for its ability to detoxify.

*Take as many as possible of these nutrients in the form of whole-food complexes. Follow the directions on the bottle for dosage.

CHAPTER 8

MENTAL AND NEUROLOGICAL DISORDERS

D r. Rodolfo Llinas, a professor at New York University Medical School, discovered an aberrant chemical reaction common to depression, Parkinson's disease, obsessive-compulsive disorder, and tinnitus (ringing in the ears). But he didn't go one step further and explore the connection between brain disorders and abnormal blood chemistrics.[1] To do so would have amounted to an admission that curing brain disorders depends on improving blood chemistry rather than manipulating brain function.

The problem lies in the neuroscience researchers' focus on the brain's extracellular functions—the motions of cells, the directions in which neurotransmitters convey thoughts and feelings, the abnormal shapes of cellular brain tissue—rather than on the internal function of the brain cell. It is what is going on inside the cells that determines how a cluster of brain cells behaves. There is as yet no way of visualizing a cell's internal functions. Since, however, the capillaries deliver nutrients, hormones, and other raw materials to the cells and pick up the by-products of their metabolic functions, a blood profile gives some idea as to what is going on inside the cell.

The connection between abnormal brain function and abnormal blood chemistry is obvious. The typical blood chemistry of someone with a mental disorder shows elevated levels of such heavy metals as copper, iron, and lead; ammonia; estrogen; histamine (an indication of allergies); and in schizophrenia alien chemicals called porphyrins and kryptopyrroles. Even some nutrients, if present in such large amounts that not all of them are used, can break down into acidic toxic waste that disturbs mental function. Excessive blood levels of copper, iron, and estrogen in the cerebrospinal (intercellular) fluid in the brain are an almost sure indication that they have made their way into the neurons through leaks in their membranes.

Wastes such as ammonia, heavy metals, lactic acid, and other debris in the blood accumulate in the brain—rather than in some other organ system—when it has sustained an injury or when a key enzyme or coenzyme in the brain is missing due to a genetic defect. Fred Bookstein of the University of Michigan's Medical Center found these extraneous substances in the brains of schizophrenics.[2] Schizophrenia is also associated with fetal brain injury due to maternal viral infections, misplacement of the fetus in the uterus, difficult pregnancies, mothers and/or fathers over the age of forty, and a family history of mental illness.

Excessive blood levels of acidic wastes, heavy metals, and ammonia in the brain are most likely responsible for the swelling and redness in two areas—the corpus callosum (the thick cluster of nerve fibers that connect the two halves of the brain) and the brain's ventricles. The elevated estrogen so commonly found in individuals with mental problems may be the real reason for the aberrant chemical reactions that Llinas found.

Symptoms of fear, anxiety, and/or depression worsen existing mental disorders because they trigger the flow of the adrenal hormone cortisol. When the release of cortisol—which is intended by the body to be liberated in big doses only as a response to life-threatening situations—is prolonged because of ongoing feelings of anxiety and fear, it destroys brain cells in the hippocampus (a part of the primitive limbic system where long-term memories are stored). This explains why most schizophrenics have a smaller than normal hippocampus. Emotional and physical abuse during childhood also causes injury to this region of the brain, and these injuries can give rise to intellectual and emotional disabilities.

Energy Deficiency in the Brain Prevents Neutralization of Toxic Waste

A lack of energy is the biggest problem in brain disorder because enzymes, vitamins, and minerals can neutralize the toxic waste in brain tissue only if there is sufficient energy. An energy deficiency can be caused by an underactive thyroid. The brain generates more energy than any other organ in the body. Although the brain is only 2 percent of body weight, it uses up 60 percent of the body's glucose reserves and 25 percent of its oxygen supply in the production of energy. Because of its voracious energy needs, a shortage of glucose is more injurious to the brain than to any other organ.

Another cause of deficient energy levels in the brain is a lack of the hormone progesterone. When, because of extreme anxiety or depression, excessive levels of cortisol are circulating in the blood, there is not enough cortisol left in the adrenal glands for its conversion into progesterone. High estrogen levels also depress progesterone levels. And excessive estrogen lowers energy production by destroying glucose and oxygen. Progesterone is vital to the brain because it lessens and sometimes even eliminates the symptoms of many brain diseases (bipolar depression, schizophrenia, Parkinson's disease, epilepsy, neuritis, and migraine headaches)—in some cases only forty minutes after it is taken.

Depressed levels of glucose, of the thyroid hormone thyroxin, and of progesterone, as well as excessively high levels of estrogen are not the only reasons that diseased brains don't generate enough energy. If the oxidoreductase enzymes in the mitochondria aren't working, even higher than normal levels of thyroxin and glucose can't increase energy levels. Dr. William H. Philpott, an expert on the therapeutic use of magnetic energy, states that the stumbling block in energy production in the brain as well as the cure of mental disease with nutritional protocols is the paralysis of these enzymes. According to Philpott, the oxidoreductase enzymes can be activated by removing acidic wastes in the affected brain area with a negatively charged magnet placed on the head. (See Resources for where to find magnets.)

Besides thyroid supplements, progesterone, and magnetic energy, the nutrients that stimulate respiration (energy production) in the brain include saturated meat fats as well as vitamin B_1 (thiamin) and vitamin C (vitamin C helps produce the amino acid tyrosine, which is converted into thyroxin, the thyroid hormone). Although most people with mental disease have excess levels of copper in their blood, anyone with a copper deficiency needs to take a supplement that includes copper because, as a receptor for red light, copper plays a vital role in respiration.

Few people realize that sunlight plays an active role in the conversion of the chemical energy in the food we eat into heat energy for body function. The importance of sunlight in the brain for the production of energy is underscored by the fact that in developing countries, although coronary heart disease, cancer, and diabetes have become common (since the introduction of refined sugar, flour, soda, and canned goods), schizophrenia and depression are still rare. While the great majority of the inhabitants in these countries have given up their traditional foods, because of the tropical climate they still spend a great deal of time in the sun. It would seem then that as far as the health of the brain is concerned, sunlight for the manufacture of energy is even more important than a healthy diet.

Cellular respiration (energy production) in the brain can also benefit from a substance not ordinarily associated with the synthesis of energy, and that is glutamic acid, an amino acid. If taken in the form of L-glutamine, it can get through the brain's highly selective blood-brain barrier. (The walls of the brain's capillaries have no receptors through which glutamic acid can pass, but they do have exit points for L-glutamine.) L-glutamine produces a special, concentrated energy useful for those with or without brain disorders who suffer from inertia. It also gets rid of excess ammonia in the blood, a problem in most mental disorders. (Dr. Roger Williams recommends 1 to 4 g L-glutamine per day for schizophrenics.) There can be a downside to taking L-glutamine: being essentially glutamic acid, the amino acid in monosodium glutamate (MSG), it is highly allergy causing. For those who are allergic to it, it acts as an excitotoxin, distorting the functions of the brain's neurons by accelerating their movements. This increased speed causes the neurons to heat up, resulting in such side effects as headaches, dizziness, and restlessness.

Nutritional Therapy for Mental Disorders

Individuals with mental disorders tend to have a deficiency in the B vitamins, vitamins E and C, and such minerals as zinc, magnesium, calcium, and manganese. Magnesium and vitamin B_6 have a calming effect on the agitated brain, but magnesium has an importance of its own. This was pointed out by the French scientist M. L. Robinet in the *Bulletin of the Academy of Medicine* originally published in France back in 1934.[3] He found that more people commit suicide in regions where the magnesium content of the soil is low. But it's not only the lack of minerals in the foods grown in mineral-deficient soil that is responsible for the low magnesium levels in the bodies of those with mental disorders.

Excessive amounts of stress hormones circulating in the blood of emotionally disturbed people deplete blood magnesium levels. But when magnesium and/or other nutrients are supplied in large enough quantities—provided energy levels in the brain are sufficient—symptoms of mental disorder can disappear. Magnesium in combination with B_6 is effective in alleviating learning disabilities and emotional disorders in children. Megadoses of niacin (vitamin B_3) cures pellagra, a vitamin B_3 deficiency disease that causes such symptoms as paranoia and hallucinations, as well as elevated blood levels of porphyrins. The latter is found in the blood of schizophrenics. In 1956, Dr. J. McDonald Holmes wrote in the *British Medical Journal* about a number of studies that showed that individuals who have a deficiency of vitamin B_{12} suffer memory loss, hallucination, paranoia, and epilepsy—until they receive injections of B_{12}.[4] The B vitamins are vital to brain function because the myelin sheathing covering the neurons in the brain contains greater concentrations of B vitamins than any other tissue in the body.

Dr. Abram Hoffer, a pioneer in the holistic treatment of mental disorders, was successful in curing schizophrenia with vitamins B_3, B_6, B_{12}, and C.[5] The effectiveness of these B vitamins stems from their ability to eliminate porphyrins, the alien chemical that causes hallucinations, paranoia, and delusions in schizophrenics. Hoffer typically starts out adults with schizophrenia and/or severe depression on 3 g of B_3 in the form of niacin and an equal amount of vitamin C and goes up depending on need to as high as 22 g of niacin. Beyond that amount, he stated there was no improvement. No sooner did he make that statement than he met a woman with schizophrenia who couldn't eliminate her symptoms until she took 60 g of vitamin B_3 a day and an unspecified amount of vitamin C. In individuals with long-standing cases of schizophrenia

Hoffer included 1 to 2 g of B_1 and B_6 as well as magnesium, calcium, manganese, and zinc.

Dr. Hans Selye, famous for his books on the physiological effects of stress, believes progesterone, given its function in promoting a balanced temperament, could ease the symptoms of schizophrenia.[6] It is not surprising that in large quantities progesterone, which is known for its calming effect, can act as an anesthetic.

Vitamin C, along with niacin, picks up the "garbage" in the blood, while vitamin B_6 enables the schizophrenic to dream, an ability that is lost as the disease worsens and the thought processes dry up. B_6 may accomplish this by neutralizing the lactic acid that typically accumulates in the blood of people with mental disorders. Anxiety causes the buildup of lactic acid in the body because, like aerobic exercise, it uses up oxygen. When there is not enough oxygen, energy has to be generated anaerobically, that is, without oxygen, the by-product of which is lactic acid. By destroying excess lactic acid, vitamin B_6 has a calming effect while also activating the dream structures in the subconscious. Several other nutrients also reduce anxiety. The high alkaline content of calcium and magnesium makes lactic acid physiologically inactive, while vitamin E lowers anxiety levels by slowing the transmission of anxiety impulses as they move between the amygdala (a primitive brain structure involved in feelings of fear and aggression) and the cortex. Vitamin E also blocks the action of porphyrins, the alien chemical that causes disordered thoughts and bizarre behavior in the schizophrenic. Zinc and calcium are two other nutrients that reduce blood toxicity by lowering excessive levels of copper and lead, which are toxic to brain cells.

It's just as important to eat a metabolically appropriate and allergen-free diet (see Chapter 2) as it is to take nutritional supplements if you have a mental disorder. Mild brain disease, for example, occasional depression or a mild obsessive-compulsive disorder, may be cured by avoiding an allergy-causing food. People with all kinds of mental and neurological disorders are particularly allergic to the proteins gluten and alpha gliadin in wheat, rye, and barley, and often to the protein in other grains as well. I believe that grains eaten during pregnancy by mothers whose fetuses are allergic to wheat is the greatest single cause of brain injuries that occur during the fetal stage of human development. This agrees with the research of Dr. Chris M. Reading, an orthomolecular physician in Australia. Reading found a link between celiac disease, an inherited digestive disorder caused by intolerance to wheat gluten, and Down syndrome. He contends that if a woman whose fetus is allergic to wheat eats wheat products during pregnancy, it can cause a doubling of chromosome 21 in the fetus. The result is Down syndrome, a form of mental retardation that is caused by the extra chromosome, because it triggers the production of chemicals the body doesn't need. These clog the blood vessels, preventing the delivery of oxygen and nutrients to the brain cells. Inadequate supplies of brain "food" explain the low IQ and emotional instability of Down syndrome victims. Reading's study of eighteen children with Down syndrome substantiates his premise. It showed that a diet free of wheat products vastly improved the mental functions of these youngsters.[7]

The gluten in grain may also cause schizophrenia and depression in people allergic to it by depleting the supply of the minerals zinc, calcium, magnesium, iron, and manganese, and vitamins B_1, B_3, B_{12}, and folic acid. Mental disorders, like other degenerative diseases, probably didn't become a problem until the cultivation of wild grain plants began.[8] Thus it's not surprising that mentally disturbed people feel more balanced on a diet that emphasizes meat, vegetables, and saturated fats, and avoid food products made of grain as well as polyunsaturated oils.

Signs of the onset of schizophrenia are a change in behavior, attitude, and personal appearance that can't be explained. But this isn't always the case. The first sign of schizophrenia in Helen, a middle-aged woman who was as stable and free of complexes as anyone I know, was a hallucination, a symptom that ordinarily occurs when the disease is well advanced. Helen and her husband live on the floodplains of a small rural town north of Seattle where, along with most of the other farmers in the area, they grow tulips. One day Helen was sitting on her front porch gazing at a large field of red tulips across the street when the tulip blossoms suddenly broke off from their stems and began doing the polka. Helen recognized this vision as a symptom of schizophrenia, and the doctor confirmed her diagnosis when a blood test revealed excess kryptopyrroles in her blood and urine. (Kryptopyrroles are also referred to as the "mauve spot" because of the reddish color they give urine.) Helen's hallucinations disappeared as abruptly as they had come on, when, after hearing that schizophrenics are often allergic to wheat, and knowing that an allergy to gluten ran in her family, she gave up all wheat products. It's amazing how quickly the body returns to normal even when afflicted with a seemingly incurable disease once the offending food allergens are removed.

Depression

There is a theory supported by numerous studies that everyone has ups and downs in moods irrespective of circumstances, that our overall sense of well-being is preset by our genes. In a study by the National Health and Nutrition Examination, the state of happiness of six thousand men and women was tracked over ten years. The results showed that those who were happiest in the beginning of the study were also the happiest at the end of the ten-year study. They never seemed to be affected by misfortune for any considerable length of time. The study concluded that those who have a high set point for happiness rebound from tragedy within six months to a year, whereas unhappy people who experience a loss fall into a depression that persists over time. By the same token, unhappy people after they, say, win the lottery or get a job promotion, lose their happy feelings by the end of a year.[9] The conclusion drawn from this and similar studies is that the threshold of happiness is as genetically determined as the color of the eyes or the shape of the nose.

The studies on which this conclusion is based, however, focused on individual differences in mood. If we compare groups of people, specifically technologically advanced cultures with preliterate ones, a different scenario emerges. While unhappy individuals are common in modern society, in preindustrial cultures happiness was the rule. European and American explorers in Africa, in the Australian outback, and in the Arctic who kept diaries wrote about the continual joking and laughter among the native porters they hired to carry their luggage. Likewise, movies of the Eskimos and Australian aborigines before they adopted the ways of the Europeans reveal people who laughed together continually as they went about their daily tasks. Such consistently high levels of happiness are a phenomenon peculiar to preindustrial cultures. That they don't exist in "civilized" society suggests that the lack of a sense of well-being is a mental disorder brought on by the environment rather than an inborn personality trait. What sets the level of happiness, according to Dr. Richard Depue, a psychologist at Cornell University, is the dopamine level in the brain. He found that people who have high dopamine levels have more positive feelings than those with lower levels of dopamine. Thus a low set point of happiness, like chronic and bipolar depression, has a physical component that may reflect a genetic weakness, but the high level of happiness of preliterate peoples indicates it is not a fixed trait. With the right nutritional environment it can be "reset" upward.

A Case of Severe Depression

Victor had been depressed, suicidal, and homicidal for a year and a half and had been hospitalized four times during that period, once for sixteen days. He had recently developed an especially disturbing symptom: hallucinations. He heard a voice in his head. The voice called himself Tom. Tom would tell Victor as he was walking along a street and saw a pretty girl to kill her. On the other hand he would warn Victor not to cross a street on a red light. He didn't want Victor to be killed he said because that would mean that he, Tom, would also die. Victor was on four antipsychotic drug medications. Of all the medications, the worst one, in terms of side effects, is respiredone. This drug causes people who have been taking it a long time to behave like robots.

I recommended that Victor start with 1 g of vitamin C and 1 g of niacin (B_3) at the end of each meal and gradually work up to 3 g of niacin and 3 g of vitamin C. After he was on the latter protocol for two months, he lost all feelings of depression. His hallucinations also disappeared, so his doctor took him off respiredone. Two months later, however, Victor again felt depressed, although his hallucinations didn't recur. I upped his vitamin C intake to 4 g along with 4 g of niacin at the end of each meal. In only one week, most of his depression had vanished.

The occasional sad episodes he still experienced had to have been mild, as he was able to eliminate them through his own efforts. What worked for him, he said, was to do something he liked. He loves technology, so whenever he felt depressed, he took machines apart and then put them back together to see if they still worked. He claims this took his depression away because he found it impossible to think of his personal problems and solve a technical problem at the same time.

While Victor said he felt "mostly good," because he still had occasional bouts of sadness and, like most people with a mental disorder, elevated blood levels of heavy metals (lead, copper, cadmium, and iron), I suggested another antidepressant: a supplement containing a combination of minerals and vitamins. Its effectiveness lies in its precise quantities. Called Empowerplus, it has been highly successful in treating bipolar and severe depression.

The impressive record of this nutritional supplement has been validated by Dr. Charles Popper, a professor at Harvard Medical School and a medical doctor with a large psychiatric practice. Dr. Popper has successfully treated more than a hundred patients with this supplement (truehope.com).[10]

SUGGESTIONS FOR BIPOLAR AND SEVERE DEPRESSION AND SCHIZOPHRENIA*

➤ **Empowerplus.** Follow the directions on the label (truehope .com).

➤ **Progesterone or pregnenolone.** The excessive levels of estrogen and cortisol in people with mental disorders require treatment with calming hormones. For women, this means natural progesterone applied topically, and for men pregnenolone, 1 to 5 mg daily. Go off these hormones periodically for one week. Follow the directions on the container. Victor has slightly developed breasts, which indicates elevated levels of prolactin and estrogen. I prescribed progesterone to reduce these stress hormone levels and eliminate his swollen breasts.

➤ **Omega-3 fish oil** (400 mg capsule). Take two in the morning, two after breakfast, and one at night. This supplement is more likely to help someone with a grain-eating metabolism. When Ricardo had a severe bout of depression he saw only blackness. Omega-3 fish oil cured his depression within days.

➤ **Milk thistle for the liver.** Milk thistle is recommended when taking niacin in large doses to protect the liver and reduce estrogen levels.

➤ **Vitamin B₃** (3 to 22 g/day). It is preferable to take this vitamin in the form of niacin (see next item).

➤ **Vitamin C and niacin.** Take 3 g of vitamin C along with 3 g of niacin at meals, but start with 1 g of each nutrient and gradually work up to the dosage that is effective in reducing symptoms. If the dosage of niacin is increased, the dosage of vitamin C should be increased by the same amount.

➤ **Vitamin B₆** (250 to 1,000 mg/day).

➤ **Vitamin B₁** (100 to 3,000 mg/day).

➤ **Folic acid and vitamin B₁₂** (1,000 to 3,000 mcg/day).

➤ **Vitamin E** (1,600 to 2,000 units/day). Taking enough vitamin E can lift depression. The vitamin E may take three months to take effect, but individuals with mild depression may find it goes away in two or three days.

➤ **L-glutamine** (1 to 4 g/day). This helps alleviate the symptoms of schizophrenia.

➤ **Mineral complex including calcium, magnesium, manganese, and zinc.**

➤ **Thyroid supplements.** To increase energy production, take a thyroid supplement, preferably a glandular such as Thytrophin made by Standard Process. A synthetic form should contain T3 as well as T4.

➤ **Ginkgo biloba** (120 mg/day). Ginkgo relieves depression by increasing the flow of blood to the brain.

*Take as many as possible of these nutrients in the form of whole-food complexes. Follow the directions on the bottle for dosage.

Migraines

When Chris drove home from work in the evening, he passed by a wooded area. With the setting sun at an angle, the light streaming through the trees created alternating bands of light and darkness. Whizzing by this scene in a car, Chris couldn't avoid seeing this strobe-like pattern from the corner of his right eye. It gave him migraine headaches.

By the time Chris parked his car in the driveway and walked through the door of his house, he was seeing neon-lit circles, stars, and stripes. Fifteen minutes later the throbbing, painful ache on the left side of his head began, and on the same side of his body his muscles became paralyzed. A half hour later he couldn't see and had trouble talking. It was two hours before his migraine symptoms began to subside.

Then Chris changed jobs. He was able to take a bus to and from work, so on his way home, he could avoid the rotating bands of light and shadow by closing his eyes. But while Chris no longer had five migraines a week, the few he did have were far more severe. This told him that the strobe-light effect simply switched on symptoms that were caused by something else.

Doing some research into migraines, Chris unearthed the information that milk, citrus fruit, chocolate, alcohol, coffee, and cheese were the most frequent causes of chronic headaches. Cheese was the only one of these foods that Chris ate in appreciable quantities. He gave it up, cut down on the number of cups of coffee he drank daily, and went on the grain eater's diet, which the niacin test indicated fit his digestive requirements. He is also having acupuncture treatments. He hasn't had a migraine in over a year and a half.

A migraine, which can last anywhere from four hours to two days, occurs in two stages. In the first stage the sufferer sees lightning-like zigzags, wavy lines, and/or dark spots. This is caused by hyperactive neurons in the visual center of the brain whose blood supply has been cut off by the constriction of the blood vessels. In the second stage the blood vessels covering the skull become enlarged and the head begins to throb painfully. Speech, hearing, and muscle problems develop during this stage.

There is no lack of theories as to why migraines develop, but none have ever been proven and some have been disproven. There is an obvious explanation that accounts for both stages of migraine. That is the presence of acidic waste in the fluid surrounding the neurons in the brain and in the blood vessels in the tissue covering the skull. The fact that the blood vessels on the side of the head where the second stage of migraines occur become enlarged and painful suggests the presence of an irritant in the blood.

A traditional Arab remedy for migraine headaches points up what this irritant is. The Arabs place a clove of garlic under the skin in the region of the temple. As soon as a pocket of pus develops under the garlic, the blood vessels shrink back to their normal size, and the headache disappears. The garlic draws out the pus from the blood in the dilated vessels. Pus is a sign of infection and contains phagocytes, which try to destroy the bacteria responsible for the infection. The bacteria wouldn't have proliferated to the extent that the phagocyte immune cells intervened if there was not enough acid waste in the blood for them to feed on. A migraine, then, is caused by acidic waste that, in providing food for bacteria, causes an infection that is painful because it inflames the blood vessels.

An effective treatment for migraine headaches was developed by an otologist, Dr. Miles Atkinson. Atkinson described the results of his vitamin B therapy. B complex, particularly B_3, helped maintain normal dilation in the brain's blood vessels in his patients suffering from migraine headaches.[11] He made this discovery quite by accident. His patients with gastrointestinal problems who took the bacterium *Lactobacillus acidophilus* (commonly found in yogurt) not only got relief from their intestinal problems, but the patients who had migraine headaches noticed that some of their migraine symptoms had disappeared as well. Atkinson came to the conclusion that by replenishing the bacterial colonies in the intestines that aid in the manufacture of the B vitamins, the brain was supplied with enough vitamin B to normalize the dilation of the blood vessels covering the skull. (He also gave vitamin B injections and prescribed oral B.) Another possibility is that the friendly bacteria in the yogurt destroyed the harmful bacteria that were causing the painful swelling of the blood vessels.

Individuals with injuries in the visual center of the brain get migraines if they eat foods their digestive systems can't handle or if they react to airborne particles such as pollen or the scent of perfume. These incompatible factors cause acids to form that accumulate near the brain injury. Migraine sufferers are known to react to coffee, tea, alcohol, wheat and other grain products, red wine, chocolate, citrus fruit, cheese, chain smoking, and pollen. Avoiding these foods and air pollutants like cigarette smoke and pollen also normalizes the thyroid so that energy levels can increase enough to eliminate the metabolic wastes and toxins that trigger migraines. Migraine sufferers, like people with other mental disorders, usually do best on a diet high in meat protein and relatively low in carbohydrates.

Migraine headaches in women may turn out to be the cloud with the silver lining. A new study reveals that women who have migraines experience less cognitive decline than women who don't have them.[12]

SUGGESTIONS FOR MIGRAINE HEADACHES*

➤ **Niacin test for metabolic type and food allergens** (see Chapter 2). If you have a balanced metabolism and therefore can digest all kinds of protein, choose a red meat diet and limit carbohydrate intake.

➤ **Thyroid supplements.** Take a glandular such as Thytrophin (made by Standard Process). If you take a synthetic form of thyroxin, take a supplement containing the active T3 as well as T4. See Chapter 5, Thyroid Problems, for other causes of hypothyroidism.

➤ **Butterbur.** This is the most effective herb for migraines. It improves blood flow in the brain. For those with severe migraine headaches that last more than a week, taking one capsule a day of feverfew along with one capsule of butterbur is a highly effective preventative.

➤ **Progesterone.** Choose natural progesterone in the form of cream applied where blood vessels are close to the skin, such as the neck, the wrist, and inside the elbows. Follow the directions on the container. In addition, skip it for one week every so often.

➤ **Vitamin E** (400 to 800 units a day). Vitamin E bolsters energy production and eliminates free radicals.

➤ **Omega-3 fats and oil.** Omega-3, good for depression, is found in green, leafy vegetables; eggs; saltwater fish, particularly mackerel, salmon, anchovies, and sardines; and omega-3 supplements.

➤ **Air cleaner.** Use an ionizer with an ozone maker to clear the air of allergens, bacteria, molds, and toxic particles. (See Resources.)

> **Acupuncture.** This prevents migraine headaches in almost 60 percent of the sufferers who use it.
> **B complex.** Take a B complex capsule containing 100 mg each of B_1, B_2, and B_3 three times a day. If you don't get significant relief, take additional B_3—up to 3,000 mg/day.

*Take as many as possible of these nutrients in the form of whole-food complexes. Follow the directions on the bottle for dosage.

Parkinson's Disease

Parkinson's disease (PD) usually develops between the ages of fifty and sixty-nine. In cases where the cause is pesticides, asbestos, or other airborne chemicals, symptoms often appear decades after exposure.

Carl is convinced he developed Parkinson's as a result of the job he had as a young man spraying polyurethane foam over metal frame house structures. The swirling particles of white polyurethane, confined in an old airplane hangar, became so thick, Carl said, that it looked like a snow blizzard. Working without a mask, Carl breathed in this powerful petrochemical for two years during his eight-hour workday. Thirty-five years later at the age of seventy he was diagnosed with PD.

For seven years before his diagnosis, Carl was presymptomatic. In the beginning his only symptoms were stiffened legs after a long walk and hands that were perpetually cold. Two years later he developed a tremor in his left arm, and his handwriting became so small that it couldn't be read without a magnifying glass. This was followed by his inability, when in a crowd of people, to focus on what was going on. It was obvious that he had tuned out when his eyes glazed over.

Wary of the long-term effects of taking L-dopamine, he refused it. Instead he went on a grain eater's diet. He also has weekly acupuncture treatments, which he believes is principally responsible for halting the progression of the disease. Carl's symptoms have not worsened during the two and a half years he has been on this protocol.

In Parkinson's disease, communication between the two regions of the brain involved in speech and coordination—the substantia nigra and the striatum—is cut off. This separation is due to the destruction of the dopamine cells that carry messages back and forth between these two regions. Dopamine cells die out when they are exposed to inflamed cells in the substantia nigra. Once there are not enough dopamine cells to coordinate the functions between the substantia nigra and the striatum, the symptoms of Parkinson's disease emerge: tremors, lack of coordination, stiffness, and speech problems.

Research studies show that a major cause of Parkinson's is the inability to digest animal fat protein, particularly red meat. The January 1999 issue of *Movement Disorders* reported a study in which 103 patients were compared with a control group of the same size.[13] The study found that individuals who ate the most meat were 300 percent more likely to develop PD. In another study in Brazil, thirty-one PD patients with a deficiency in vitamin B_2 (riboflavin) were given 30 mg of B_2 every eight hours and forbidden to eat red meat. After six months, the patients' motor capacity had increased nearly 30 percent.[14]

Exposure to pesticides and herbicides has also been implicated in PD. A startlingly high percentage of professional field hockey players have PD. There is speculation that the cause is the grassy soccer fields they play on. There is not a weed growing on any of these soccer fields—because they are heavily sprayed with chemicals.

SUGGESTIONS FOR PARKINSON'S DISEASE*

➤ **Intravenous glutathione.** Glutathione is a powerful antioxidant that destroys free radicals. It relieves many neurodegenerative diseases in addition to Parkinson's, including Alzheimer's, multiple sclerosis, fibromyalgia, and cystic fibrosis.

➤ **N-acetyl cysteine and organic whey protein.** These supplements enhance the body's production of glutathione.

➤ **Vitamin B_2** (riboflavin) (15 to 50 mg/day).

➤ **A vegetarian diet for those who can't digest meat protein, and for meat eaters as little meat fat as possible.**

---

*Take as many nutrients as possible in the form of whole-food complexes. For usage, follow the directions on the label.

Alzheimer's Disease

Before Rebecca developed Alzheimer's she suffered from atherosclerosis. She said that the hardening of her arteries started when she was a child. At the age of four she had severe pains in her feet; in her teens the pain had crept up into her legs. Then in her early forties she developed chest pains. At the age of seventy, she was showing symptoms of Alzheimer's. I believe the same condition that caused the hardening of Rebecca's arteries when she was a child also hardened the protein strands in her brain in older age.

Modern science views Alzheimer's and cardiovascular disease as two different pathologies presumably because calcified plaques that trigger the development of blood clots adhere to the arteries whereas the beta-amyloid plaques that characterize Alzheimer's float in the watery lymphlike fluid surrounding the neurons in the brain.

However, before the onset of Alzheimer's, the protein strands inside the neurons that extend beyond the neurons' cellular membranes perform the same function for the brain as arteries do for the rest of the body: they transport materials to and from their destination. Furthermore, the protein strands in the brain harden (and are deposited in amyloid plaques) just as arteries harden. It makes sense that both the arteries in the circulatory system and the protein strands that grow through the brain's neurons are exposed to acidic wastes—the protein strands from the acidic by-products of the metabolic processes that go on inside the brain, and the arteries from the acidic waste by-products the blood picks up from the various organ systems in the body.

The efforts of mainstream medicine to eliminate amyloid plaque in the brains of Alzheimer's patients, if successful, might very well interfere with normal brain function. The protease enzymes that cut the protein strands into segments so they can be deposited in amyloid plaques are programmed to get rid of old protein strands. Amyloid plaques may therefore act as waste deposit sites for protein strands that have outworn their usefulness. The fact that these plaques are held together by a protective structure of metals and a waxy, cholesterol-like substance reinforces this possibility and makes the prevention of amyloid plaques tantamount to interfering with the brain's waste disposal system. The most convincing evidence against eliminating these plaques is that *only those beta-amyloid plaques that have become inflamed destroy brain cells.*

The important question then is how amyloid plaques become inflamed in the first place. Here is a likely scenario. The highly selective blood-brain barrier in the brain's micro blood vessels develops leaks. These leaks exude harmful substances such as acid waste, which depletes oxygen. In the absence of oxygen amyloid plaques become inflamed. When brain cells come in contact with these inflamed plaques, they also become inflamed and die off. With the death of a critical number of brain cells, Alzheimer's becomes symptomatic.

One plausible reason that acidic wastes inflame amyloid plaques is that a brain injury has disabled the respiratory machinery so that there isn't enough energy to dispose of acidic waste debris in the brain. Other causes were discovered in a study conducted by Kunihiro Uryu, Ph.D., at the University of Pennsylvania's Center for Neurodegenerative Diseases.[15] The study found that both mild repetitive head injuries and serious single head injuries increase the chances of developing Alzheimer's. The study found that, in the case of men, serious head injuries increase the chances of developing Alzheimer's in old age. Of the 1,800 male marine and navy veterans who were the subjects of the study, 548 had suffered a head injury and 1,228 had not. While family history, tobacco, and alcohol abuse played a small role in the disease, the veterans with serious head injuries—especially those who were unconscious for more than twenty-four hours—and mild repetitive injuries had four times the risk of developing Alzheimer's or other types of dementia as opposed to the men who had suffered no head injuries. No matter where in the brain the head injuries occurred, they resulted decades later in some form of dementia—particularly Alzheimer's—rather than some other brain disease such as Parkinson's or obsessive-compulsive disorder. According to the research scientists involved in the study, the symptoms of Alzheimer's—increased free-radical damage and the proliferation of amyloid plaques—are more likely to occur in areas of the brain, such as the hippocampus, that are involved in the most complicated tasks.

Physical trauma and acid particles from putrefied food waste are hardly the only inflammatory factors that are likely to lead to Alzheimer's. Heavy metals in flu shots, such as thimersol (a mercury-derived preservative) and aluminum, are also suspect. Hugh Fudenberg, M.D., a leading immunologist and founder and director of research at the Neuro Immuno Therapeutics Research Foundation, Inman, South Carolina, states that the chances of getting Alzheimer's is ten times higher if an individual has had five consecutive annual flu shots.[16]

Nutritional Supplements for Alzheimer's Disease

The formation of amyloid plaques begins when enzymes cut the protein strands that extend outward from the neurons into shorter strands. These short strands of protein form clusters and are covered with a metal framework and a sticky, waxy substance. As the by-products of the brain cells' metabolism, it is not surprising that everyone has some amyloid plaques, but Alzheimer's victims have many more.

Research shows that testosterone in men and estradiol, a form of estrogen, in women protect the neurons from injury and reduce the number of amyloid plaques in the brain.[17] The role of these hormones in preventing neuron inflammation suggests that like vitamin E, they increase brain oxygen levels. The oxygen neutralizes the acid waste that is responsible for inflaming the neurons. Without inflammation, Alzheimer's doesn't happen.

Because a deficiency in estradiol and testosterone increases the chances of Alzheimer's, if you don't have optimal levels of these hormones you should take them—testosterone with pregnenolone if you are a man, and estradiol with progesterone if you are a woman. Take only the natural form of these hormones. Other protocols that are beneficial are thyroid supplements (preferably a natural one such as Thytrophin) to stimulate sluggish thyroid function, CoQ-10, and vitamin D₃. (A British study published in the *Journal of Geriatric Psychology and Neurology* and that appeared online consisted of 1,766 people divided into groups according to their vitamin D blood levels. The lower the level of vitamin D, the more cognitively impaired they were. Compared to the group with the highest level of vitamin D, people in the low-end group were 2.3 times as likely to suffer from dementia.[18])

A research study has found that the best treatment for Alzheimer's is lithium. A National Institutes of Health (NIH) report, cited in the journal *Nature*, found in studies of mice and human cells that lithium blocked an enzyme vital to the formation of amyloid plaques and "neurofibrillary tangles." This blockage thus succeeds in preventing their accumulation. [19]

Many health-care professionals still don't seem to be aware of vitamin E's ability to delay the worsening of Alzheimer's symptoms. One study reveals that in middle-aged and older animals, supplements of vitamin E prevented the conversion of the protein strands in the brain into beta-amyloid plaques.[20] Another study showed that humans with Alzheimer's as well as animals can profit from vitamin E. Directed by Mary Sano, an associate professor of clinical neuropsychology at Columbia University, the study found that patients who took high doses of vitamin E delayed having to go into a nursing home by seven months.[21] By making more oxygen available, vitamin E helps to heal inflamed tissues. Additional oxygen can also prevent the inflammatory process from happening in the first place. Vitamin E could also prevent the inflammation of protein strands by clearing away toxic acidic waste in the intercellular fluid surrounding the neurons before it gets the inflammatory process going. Like vitamin C, vitamin E removes toxic waste, but unlike vitamin C it's fat soluble so it can go through the double-layered fatty membrane surrounding the neurons where the main portion of these protein strands are located.

Vitamin E is most effective in delaying the onset of Alzheimer's because by oxygenating brain tissue it neutralizes the acidic condition that causes inflammation. Another effective anti-inflammatory supplement is huperzine A, a type of club moss that has been used for thousands of years by the Chinese to treat inflammation. Huperzine A can cross the blood-brain barrier and in animal experiments has been shown to soothe, protect, and even regenerate neurons.

Maintaining cellular energy is the best way to protect the brain cells from the toxicity of acidic waste. Besides thyroid supplements and vitamin E to normalize thyroid function, and natural progesterone to ensure a balance of steroid hormone function, coenzyme Q-10 (CoQ-10) and acetyl-L-carnitine help maintain energy levels in the brain cells: CoQ-10 by transporting electrons that are involved in respiration, and acetyl-L-carnitine by transporting fats into cells where it is burned to produce cellular energy.

SUGGESTIONS FOR ALZHEIMER'S DISEASE*

➤ **Thyroid.** Look for Thytrophin (made by Standard Process) or a synthetic supplement that contains T3 as well as T4. (See Resources.)

➤ **Progesterone.** Use a natural topical cream. Follow the directions on the label. Go off it periodically for one week.

➤ **CoQ-10** (150 mg/day). Choose Ubiquinol, the active form.

➤ **Acetyl-L-carnitine** (500 to 1,500 mg/day).

➤ **NADH (nicotinamide adenine dinucleotide)** (5 to 10 mg/day). NADH (the H stands for hydrogen), found in the muscle tissue of poultry and cattle, relieves Parkinson's, Alzheimer's, chronic fatigue, and depression.

➤ **High-intensity light.** Spend one-half hour to one hour every morning in high-intensity light to restore the mitochondria's ability to manufacture energy.

➤ **B-complex capsule.** Take a B complex three times daily to reduce homocysteine levels. Excess homocysteine turns into acid waste and destroys brain cells. According to Robert Clark, M.D., of Oxford University, people with low blood levels of folic acid, B_{12}, and B_6 have the highest levels of homocysteine and are three to four times more likely to develop Alzheimer's disease.

➤ **Vitamin C** (1,000 mg/day).

➤ **Omega-3 fats and oils.** Omega-3, found in saltwater fish and green, leafy vegetables, has an anti-inflammatory effect that helps offset the inflammatory effect of omega-6 polyunsaturated oils.

➤ **Removal of silver/mercury dental amalgams** has been known to stop the progression of Alzheimer's, but the removal must be done according to the system devised by Hal Huggins, D.D.S.[22]

*Take as many of these nutrients as possible in the form of whole-food complexes. Follow the directions on the label.

Epilepsy

While little is known about epilepsy, electroencephalograms (EEGs) give a clue as to its underlying cause by showing that the brain waves in epileptics, even when the brain is not undergoing a seizure, contain an excess of electrical activity. (Medications such as Dilantin and Depakote prevent tonic-clonic, or grand mal, seizures by reducing electricity in the brain.) Electricity is generated by the overactivity of neurons that have become inflamed. Inflammation—from exposure to toxic waste, estrogen, glutamate, heavy metals—causes the electrons orbiting around the nucleus inside the neurons to speed up so that they generate too much electricity. Excessive electrical activity in turn heats up the neurons, causing them to spin so fast that they can no longer communicate with other cells. The degree to which the neurons "go crazy"— that is, whether symptoms will be partial seizures (petite mals) or will escalate into tonic-clonic (grand mal) seizures—depends on how inflamed the neurons are.

I suspect that the pathology of epilepsy is no different from that of most other neurological disorders since the neurons in particular areas of the brain in Parkinson's disease, obsessive-compulsive disorders, tinnitus, and depression, like those in epilepsy, are overactive. That the symptoms presented constitute epilepsy rather than one of these other mental disorders is due to the location of the brain injury.

When epilepsy is accompanied by frequent headaches, food allergies are suspect. This could happen if injured areas in the brain are exposed to the acidic wastes from food allergens. This would trigger seizures by causing the neurons to spin out of control.

The Ketogenic Diet for Epilepsy

In an impressive number of cases, mostly children, of those whose epilepsy could not be controlled with drug medications, the ketogenic diet has lessened or prevented tonic-clonic (grand mal) seizures. This is a diet in which four times more fat than protein and carbohydrates combined is eaten. Saturated fats such as butter, cream, cheese, bacon, fatty pork, and beef fat are most effective. Saturated fat is said to prevent seizures because fat rather than sugar is burned as energy, producing ketones, which, when absorbed into the blood, calm the nerves, thereby lessening the severity of seizures or stopping them altogether. Saturated fats may also act by patching up the holes and tears in brain cellular membranes through which toxic waste infiltrates the cells.

Medical research is based on the premise that cures for brain disease depend on discovering how the brain functions. But the thrill of discovering unknown brain functions—for example, the way neurons transmit or store memory or the amount of fuel the brain uses up during problem solving—clouds the real issue: how to heal the brain abnormalities that cause mental disorders. This healing depends on three factors: individual differences in food metabolism and eating habits; the condition of the thyroid and respiratory brain machinery; and nutritional and enzyme deficiencies in the brain. When any or all of these factors cause the brain to malfunction, since the brain controls the thought processes, regulates mood, and coordinates movement, a variety of behavioral and muscular disorders follow.

SUGGESTIONS FOR EPILEPSY*

➤ **Progesterone.** Progesterone helps prevent seizures. Buy natural progesterone, in the form of a topical cream, and apply where blood vessels are close to the skin, for example, the neck and wrist. Follow the directions on the label. Go off the hormone periodically for a week. According to chemist Ray Peat, Ph.D., progesterone works in three stages: it soothes, then protects, and finally causes the brain cells to regenerate.[23]

➤ **A ketogenic diet.** Follow a ketogenic diet, in which four times as much saturated fat as protein and carbohydrates is consumed, that is, 4 g of fat to 1 g of protein and carbohydrate foods. (See Resources for additional information.)

➤ **Coconut oil.** All of this supersaturated fat is used as a fuel to produce energy. It is therefore the best type of fatty acid for an epileptic individual on the ketogenic diet.

continued

➤ **Vitamin B$_6$.** Seizures in babies and small children have been relieved with 50 to 100 mg/day of B$_6$. For adults, 200 to 300 mg/day have been effective.

➤ **Vitamin D** (1,000 units/day). Vitamin D helps one out of three people who take it.

➤ **Magnesium** (700 mg broken up into three doses daily). In combination with B$_6$, magnesium seems to have a calming effect on injured brain cells.

➤ **Taurine** (1 to 5 g/day).

➤ **L-tyrosine** (500 mg three times daily).

➤ **Avoid polyunsaturated oils**, which become rancid, lowering thyroid function and poisoning the respiratory machinery (mitochondria) in the cells.

*Take as many of these nutrients as possible in the form of whole-food complexes. For dosage, follow the directions on the label.

CHAPTER 9

LUNG DISORDERS

The digestive tract is injured by the chemicals in the processed food it breaks down, the kidneys by the toxins they filter from the blood—and the lungs by the air pollutants that diffuse through their air sacs. Thus the first consideration in ensuring the health of the lungs is to breathe in clean air. The second is to increase the volume of air you take in. Maximizing air intake has the same effect on the lungs as exercise has on the muscles: it strengthens them and by doing so improves their function. Diet, nutritional supplements, and herbs are also beneficial to the health of the lungs.

Asthma

Christina is an example of how a supplement miraculously cured a major lung problem. Now forty-five, Christina had immigrated with her husband and children to the United States from the Dominican Republic twenty years ago. A few months after they arrived, Christina had an asthmatic attack. It was so acute that her husband called 911, and she was taken to the hospital by ambulance. That was just the first of a series of asthmatic attacks that led to her hospitalization fifty times in a five-year period. In between these attacks she struggled day to day with her asthmatic condition, wheezing after the least physical exertion, including picking up a toy, making a bed, or doing the dishes. Her doctors considered her disabled enough to authorize Medicaid payments for a full-time housekeeper.

Christina's life took an unexpected turn for the better thanks to a chance encounter. Sitting in the waiting room of her doctor's office, a fellow patient told her about a folk remedy for asthma used in the rural areas of Puerto Rico: grapefruit juice mixed with peeled and finely chopped aloe vera, a cactus-like plant found in supermarkets and grocery stores in Hispanic neighborhoods. Christina was open to this suggestion, she said, because the side effects of the anti-inflammatory steroid hormones she was taking—painful joints, the swelling of her entire body, and dizziness—were worse than the drowning sensation she felt when she was having an asthmatic attack and couldn't catch her breath. The same day she was told about this herbal concoction Christina made a five-gallon container of it. She has not had an asthmatic attack since she began drinking the aloe vera mixture sixteen years ago.

Before she began using aloe vera, Christina, like most people with asthma, used antispasmodic inhalers when she had trouble breathing. Just a few sprays open up the air passages in the lungs. But those asthma patients who rely most heavily on inhalers run twice the risk of dying. Two studies conducted in New Zealand and Canada documented the dangers of bronchodilators.[1] These statistics became real to me when Jacob, a friend, died from overuse of an inhaler. Jacob pulled his inhaler out of his pocket whenever he wheezed. One day it didn't open up his breathing passages. He had used it once too often. With no one around to rush him to a hospital, he died.

The high mortality rate of regular users of inhalers indicates they can lose their effectiveness. The inhaler (bronchodilator) is also dangerous because it gives sufferers a false sense of wellness. Relieved when the inhaler has given them their breath back, they don't realize that their bronchial tubes and alveoli (air sacs) are still inflamed.

Doctors have become increasingly concerned about lung inflammation that is chronic in individuals who have frequent asthma attacks. Not only does inflammation make the lungs more prone to future attacks, but it eventually causes lung tissue to deteriorate. This has changed the medical profession's perception of asthma from a disease that strikes periodically and is largely a problem during childhood to one that is chronic and lasts a lifetime. The current practice is to recommend medication—corticosteroid hormones—on a continuing basis for moderate and severe asthmatics.

The longtime use of such hormones has severe side effects. While they reduce inflammation, they also cause weight gain, dark moods, and anger, and they can stunt growth. Side effects in adults are elevated blood pressure and blood sugar, cataracts, and osteoporosis. So while prednisone and cortisone have saved many from immediate death, their constant use reduces the quality of life and lays the foundation for degenerative disease. The problem for asthmatics in the long run, then, is perhaps less the acute breathing problems than the chronically inflamed bronchial tubes and air sacs that force the use of corticosteroid (stress) hormones.

Causes of Asthma

While allergic reactions are undoubtedly related to defects in the adrenal and insulin-producing glands, it is not by chance that the lungs become the site of immune reactions rather than other organs. Any number of factors can sensitize the lungs to normal airborne substances, including injury.

Lung injury can occur during prenatal development. The croup, bronchitis, and asthma my brother and I had when we were young and passed on to our children were most likely the result of injury to our fetal lungs. My mother, who smoked through both her pregnancies, inhaled the smoke from four packs of cigarettes each day.

Air pollution is also a factor in asthma. A study by allergist Dr. E. M. Drost found that air pollutants destroy the elastic fibers in the alveoli.[2] But even when air pollutants don't appear to damage the lungs, the lungs' immune cells, unless supplied with sufficient enzymes to neutralize airborne pollutants as they pass through the air sacs, will react to toxic particles the same way they react to an injury—by triggering the release of histamines.

Statistics published in an article in the May 2000 issue of *The Atlantic Monthly* by Ellen Ruppel Shell rate the borough of the Bronx in New York City as the asthma capital of the United States with three times more hospitalization of asthma patients there than in any other area in the United States. Shell attributes this asthma epidemic to the fact that the Bronx is the hub of trains and trucks delivering cargo from all parts of the country, and to the fact that Interstate 95—the major truck route from Florida to Maine—cuts through the middle of the Bronx.[3]

The relationship between highly trafficked areas and astronomical rates of asthma are a warning that families with asthmatic children should avoid living in areas where there are major freeways and frequent traffic jams. When an acquaintance of mine, a teenage girl, moved from the Bronx to the upper west side of Manhattan—some would say from the frying pan into the fire—her asthmatic attacks became less threatening apparently because she had moved away from Interstate 95. Since, however, air pollution is endemic in all parts of the country, the only way you can breathe relatively pure air is to buy an air cleaner, preferably with an ozone maker, which destroys harmful bacteria and molds. (See Resources for where to find an air cleaner.)

Toxicity inside the body as well as in the environment can cause asthma. Acidic toxic gases enter the bloodstream from the colon and are carried by the blood to the liver and kidneys for detoxification. But when these two detoxifying organs are already overburdened with toxins, the latter are passed on to the lungs.

That acidic waste in the form of gas is a factor in all asthmatic lung problems is confirmed by the discovery of Dr. Benjamin Glaston, associate professor of pediatric pulmonary medicine at the University of Virginia. According to Dr. Glaston, an asthmatic's breath is 1,000 times more acidic than normal breath. Normal breath is slightly alkaline with a pH of 7.4, the same pH as the blood, but when asthmatics are sick and wheezing, their breath pH drops to 5—into the acidic range.

Asthmatics and High Blood Sugar

For asthmatics who have low blood sugar, an attack becomes more likely when blood sugar levels suddenly spike, thus eliciting a strong insulin response that causes the blood sugar to take a sharp plunge. Excessively high blood insulin levels grab the attention of the immune system, which interprets these hyped-up insulin secretions as a fight-or-flight reaction against disease-causing germs. The lungs' immune cells help mobilize the lungs against its "enemies"—normal particles such as pollen, mites, or cat dander—by triggering the release of histamine. Histamine causes blood to flow to the lung tissue just as it does when there is an injury or infection. This inflames the bronchial tubes and alveoli (air sacs). When inflamed bronchial tubes become constricted, an asthmatic attack occurs.

That high insulin levels in response to elevated blood sugar are a major factor in asthmatic attacks is confirmed by the fact that type 1 diabetics who have low insulin levels don't get asthma or any other type of allergic reaction.

To protect the lungs against immune reactions that can occur as a result of malfunctioning insulin and adrenal glands (the adrenal cortex in asthmatics doesn't secrete enough cortisone), supplements of pancreatic enzymes and adrenal extract should be taken. Vitamin C (it is stored in the adrenals) also helps normalize the function of these glands. Harry N. Holmen, Ph.D., describes the relief of eighteen asthmatic patients who were given vitamin C supplements.[4]

Avoiding the consumption of white flour and white sugar is the most important factor in keeping blood sugar levels from escalating and, by doing so, maintaining normal insulin levels. Honey is a good substitute for white sugar if it is unfiltered and unheated because it contains levulose, a type of sugar that, unlike dextrose, maltose, and sucrose, is absorbed into the blood so slowly it doesn't cause blood sugar levels to rise excessively. Dark honey is preferable because it contains the most levulose. Lightly cooked white potatoes are also effective in maintaining normal blood sugar levels—contrary to what you hear and read about them. Starch is ordinarily converted into sugar in the blood, causing blood sugar levels to rise. The exception is the starch in potatoes. That's because potatoes aren't digested. They break down by the process of fermentation in the large intestine, where there is no insulin to convert the starch into sugar. As a result, white potatoes actually lower blood sugar.

Nutritional Treatments for Asthma

The asthmatic's problems with acidic blood and breath as well as toxic gas in the lungs call for the reduction of acidic waste not only in the lungs but in the entire body. The high alkaline content of celery and dandelion leaf juice neutralizes some of the acidity in the lungs and the rest of the body. Celery, carrot, and endive juice clears mucus and acidic debris from the lungs. It also eliminates carbon dioxide that the alveoli in the lungs are too constricted to exhale. Since asthma is often triggered by a backup of toxic waste that flows into the lungs from the liver, kidneys, and colon—waste that is the product of incomplete digestion of food in the stomach and small intestine—these organs need to be detoxified. Potato and carrot juice are good general cleansers of all these organs, particularly the liver, while the chlorine in cabbage cleans the debris from the mucous membranes in the stomach.

Detoxification of the colon is the most effective means of preventing asthmatic attacks because it is in the colon that acidic waste matter gives off toxic gas that diffuses from the colon to the liver or kidneys and then onto the lungs. My students at City College who are from the Caribbean islands describe an old folk remedy—a dose of castor oil once a month—which proves that by removing toxins from the colon, asthmatic attacks can be prevented. When asked why this remedy works, they reply, "Clogged colon, clogged lungs." The fact that garlic often heals respiratory and intestinal disorders at the same time supports the contention that detoxifying the colon clears up the lungs. Professor E. Roos of St. John's hospital in Freiburg, Germany, used garlic to cure a patient of diarrhea. Not only was her intestinal function normalized, but the swelling and redness of her tubercular lungs also went down.

Asthma and other lung diseases are associated with a green vegetable deficiency. The healing of a severe asthmatic with a "green" drink is an example. Myron Cheminrow, a vegetarian and long-distance runner, teaches children who are homebound because of illness. He had a student, age twelve, who had asthma so severe he was on seven different medications. Kevin spent more time in the hospital than at home and was too drugged to do much of anything, let alone his schoolwork. A bright boy with an above-average IQ, Kevin was three grade levels behind in reading and could hardly hold a pencil in his hand. Both mother and son were desperate enough to follow any nutritional advice that Myron had to offer.

He recommended what Kevin referred to as "a whole plateful of vitamin pills" as well as four teaspoons of green powder made up of freeze-dried vegetables in juice or water. Myron also attached a water filter to the water line under the kitchen sink and to the faucet in the bathtub because Kevin got hives from the chlorine in the water. At Myron's suggestion, Kevin's mother bought an air cleaner. This regimen brought Kevin back to life. He is now on only one drug, can run and play after being an invalid for three years, and writes legibly for the first time since he began home schooling. Myron asked Kevin's mother what, out of everything he recommended, helped Kevin most. She answered without hesitating: "The freeze-dried green vegetable powder."

Why is it that green vegetables, but not red, purple, orange, or white, have worked miracles for people with asthma and other lung conditions? Several studies show that pregnant women who eat lots of green, leafy vegetables and fish during pregnancy are less likely to have asthmatic children. Fish and green vegetables are two out of three solid foods—the other is eggs—that contain omega-3 fatty acid. Chlorophyll, the green coloring that is found in large amounts in dark green leafy vegetables, is the repository for omega-3 fatty acid. Unsaturated omega-3 fatty acid is one of the building blocks of cell membranes. The role of omega-3 fatty acid in assuring the integrity of the cell membrane explains why omega-3 in green vegetables and fish is so healing to the asthmatic's lungs. Strengthening the membranes of the lung cells helps prevent inflammatory histamines from entering the holes in weak cell membranes and triggering an attack of asthma.

Asthma has also been associated with an immature immune system. Protecting children against germs by using antibacterial agents, immunization shots, and antibiotics may prevent a host of childhood ailments, but it doesn't give children's immune cells the exposure to harmful bacteria, viruses, and other parasites they need in order to learn the difference between disease-causing germs and harmless or friendly ones. Paoli Matricardi, an immunologist in the Italian Air Force, conducted a study comparing two groups of male cadets, 240 subjects in all.[5] Allergies were rare among those who had been exposed to three common foodborne pathogens, while the group that had no exposure to these pathogens had elevated allergic responses. Supporting these findings is the well-known fact that children living in rural areas of developing countries who are exposed to parasites and bacteria rarely develop asthma.

The modern world is a breeding ground for asthma wherever factories are built or processed foods are introduced. Medical interventions also contribute to the increase in asthma. Antibiotics, by killing off harmful bacteria, prevent the immune system from learning what germs it must guard against. They also give the immune system the impression that it is no longer needed to defend the body against disease-causing microbes. Another downside to drug medications when used routinely is their destruction of coenzymes (vitamins and minerals) that assist enzymes in carrying out lung function. Chemical food additives also destroy lung enzymes.

But drug medications and other man-made chemicals are most dangerous because, not being natural substances, the body has not developed the mechanisms for eliminating them. They remain in the body—unless a special effort is made to eliminate them (see Chapter 1)—forming toxic residues that acidify the pH factor of the blood and other body fluids and clog and inflame the blood and lymph vessels near the lungs. This prevents the delivery of digested food particles and oxygen to lung cells. Starving lung cells develop injuries that make them sensitive to airborne particles.

Genetics also plays a role in asthma. Carole Ober, a professor of human genetics at the University of Chicago, has found a genetic basis for the 15 percent of Hutterites (a religious sect living in South Dakota) who have asthma.[6] But because they live in rural areas where they are exposed to parasites from farm animals, where fast-food restaurants are not accessible, and where all infants have been breast-fed for at least nine months, asthma never becomes a serious problem. It is so mild that many of the Hutterites didn't even know they had asthma before she told them.

SUGGESTIONS FOR ASTHMA*

➤ **Avoid all refined carbohydrates.**
➤ **Test for your metabolic type and for food allergies and follow an appropriate diet.**
➤ **Green powder.** Take four to six teaspoons a day in juice or water. Freeze-dried green vegetables build healthy cellular membranes.
➤ **Omega-3 fatty acid capsules** (1,000 to 2,000 mg/day). Take less, for example, 500 mg/day, if you are a meat eater.
➤ **Raw adrenal extract.** Take two tablets of freeze-dried capsules a day.

➤ **Pancreatic enzyme tablets.** Take two to three tablets with each meal; this is only for individuals who are thirty years old or over.

➤ **Vitamin A** (25,000 to 50,000 units a day). It helps build healthy mucous membranes and is an immune system booster.

➤ **Vitamin D** (1,000 to 2,000 units/day).

➤ **Vitamin E** (400 to 1,200 units/day). Vitamin E oxygenizes the asthmatic's oxygen-deficient lungs.

➤ **Vitamin C** (1,000 mg two to six times per day). Do this for a few weeks periodically to detoxify allergens in the blood.

➤ **Vitamin B$_6$** (100 to 200 mg/day). B$_6$ acts as an antihistamine.

➤ **Garlic.** Take two to three capsules with each meal to clear out the lungs and colon.

➤ **Aloe vera.** Peel and chop finely. Add either to fruit juice or to beaten egg whites.

➤ **Melatonin.** Check with your doctor before using. A study at the Hebrew University Hadassah Medical School and Cardiopulmonary Laboratory in Israel found that melatonin administered to dogs intravenously dilated the lungs as effectively as drug medications. People with autoimmune diseases should not take melatonin.

➤ **Ginkgo biloba extract.** The first plant to grow after the atomic bombing of Hiroshima, ginkgo diminishes asthma-stimulating allergens and airborne bacteria in the blood.[7]

➤ **Ice pack.** Rub ice cubes wrapped in a dish towel on the chest, usually for a minimum of two to three hours during an asthmatic attack. This treatment gradually opens up constricted bronchial tubes and eliminates the aftermath of asthmatic attacks—wheezing.

➤ **Sea salt.** Add sea salt to warm water and place two or three drops of the solution in each nostril. This destroys the pollen and other airborne allergy-causing particles that cause wheezing and colds that can lead to asthmatic attacks.

continued

> **Cod liver oil, honey, and lemon.** Take a combination of one teaspoon of cod liver oil, one teaspoon of honey, and a few squirts of lemon mixed together once a day (an old West Indian custom).

> **Eliminate dust mites.** Place an air cleaner (see Resources) on the bed and cover with a sheet for one hour a day, or use mattresses made of organic cotton, flame-retardant wool, or natural latex. These natural products prevent the proliferation of mites by absorbing body sweat.

*Take as many of these nutrients as possible in the form of whole-food complexes. For dosage, follow the directions on the label.

Some of the factors that make certain individuals vulnerable to asthmatic attacks, such as genes, immature immune cells, and lung injuries, can't be changed. But these factors alone don't trigger asthmatic attacks. The other factors involved in asthmatic attacks can be controlled by diet or nutritional supplements. These are blood sugar levels, adrenal and insulin function, the integrity of the lungs' cellular membranes, the quality of air, and the acidic waste in the body that ends up in the lungs. Indeed, judging by the hyperacidity of the blood and breath of the asthmatic, acidic waste particles and toxic acidic gas are at the root of the chronic inflammation that turns asthma from a minor complaint, as it is among the Hutterites, into a lifelong degenerative disease that shortens life. A diet customized to fit the metabolic needs of the individual that also includes a lot of green leafy vegetables (people with a meat-eater metabolism, however, need to go easy on them) and raw, unprocessed foods is the most effective weapons against the lung inflammation that triggers asthma.

Emphysema

The two bronchial tubes, each connected to a lung, look like upside-down tree trunks from which progressively smaller branches—the bronchioles—radiate. Hanging off these bronchioles, like bunches of grapes, are millions of microscopic alveoli (air sacs) that do the work of the lungs.

Inhaled air flows into the trachea in the throat, through the bronchial tubes, into the bronchioles, and finally into the air sacs. From there it diffuses through the membranes of the air sacs into the blood vessels lining the air sacs' surface. The oxygen is then carried by the blood vessels to the cells, where it's used to produce energy and kill off unfriendly substances such as cancer cells. The waste product from energy production, carbon dioxide, takes the reverse route. Picked up by the blood vessels in the intercellular fluid surrounding the cells, it is carried by the circulating blood to the same blood vessels encircling the air sacs into which oxygen from the air sacs flows. Once inside the alveolar sacs, carbon dioxide is expelled from the lungs.

In emphysema, the deterioration of the air sacs interferes with the exchange of oxygen and carbon dioxide. Airborne pollutants such as cigarette smoke and industrial exhaust eat up oxygen in the lungs, inflaming the air sacs. Chronically inflamed air sacs eventually rupture and combine to form large air pockets. The walls of these air pockets aren't permeable enough to enable the oxygen to diffuse into the surrounding blood vessels. As a result, circulating blood, deprived of oxygen, is unable to deliver enough oxygen to the cells. Moreover, the loss of elasticity in the air sacs makes it impossible for the lungs to expel all the carbon dioxide waste-product from cellular metabolism. So the CO_2 remains trapped inside the alveoli, taking up space intended for oxygen.

The emphysema victim's scarcely moving chest swells up with the carbon dioxide that can't be exhaled. The lungs are also overloaded with oxygen that isn't being absorbed into the circulating blood. What happens to the cells that don't receive enough oxygen to satisfy their energy needs? They rob Peter to pay Paul, grabbing one oxygen atom from each carbon dioxide molecule (CO_2), and in doing so, they turn carbon dioxide into carbon monoxide (CO), a deadly compound, which further damages the air sacs (alveoli) in the lungs.

Another source of the toxins that contribute to the destruction of the alveoli in the lungs are metabolic wastes that the liver and kidneys are too overworked to process. When the liver can't detoxify poisonous gas from the colon, the latter is carried by the blood out of the liver and transported through the bloodstream to the lungs. The lungs become a dumping ground for the kidneys as well. The gaseous wastes the kidneys can't handle are also carried by the blood to the lungs. Processing these metabolic wastes is hard on the lungs because they were designed to eliminate carbon dioxide, not toxic waste. While they harbor macrophages and other white blood cells that devour germs and dust, unlike the liver and the lymph glands, the lungs can't neutralize toxic waste.

Industrial Pollutants and Lung Disease

According to the American Lung Association, in 2008, 35 million Americans now have chronic lung disease. It is now the United States' number three killer and accounts for one in six deaths. The implication in these and similar statistical research studies is that cigarette smoking is the chief culprit. However, the role that pollutants other than tobacco smoke play in lung disease should be the subject of more research studies.

The problem with focusing most research on the harmful effects of cigarette smoking is that the latter has acquired a monopoly on the public's and Congress's attention. It's the tobacco companies that have to issue a warning on their cigarette packs and whose product is highly taxed to discourage customers. This lets other air-polluting industries off the hook. They can spew pollutants into the air without having to take the consequences because the tobacco industry has taken the heat off them.

However, research studies carried out over the decades in which industrialization expanded by leaps and bounds and the automobile was introduced indicate that industrial air pollutants are even more responsible than cigarette smoking for the startling increase in emphysema, lung cancer, and asthma. Dr. Eugene Houdry, an inventor and lifetime researcher of the petroleum industry, stated that the nearly 2,000 percent increase in lung cancer between 1914 and 1975 corresponds with the increase in gasoline consumption.[8] Strengthening the connection between lung cancer and the burning of petroleum are statistics showing that lung cancer decreased 35 percent between 1941 and 1945 during World War II, when gasoline was rationed. This establishes vehicular exhaust as a major factor in lung cancer and brings up the possibility that if cars hadn't been invented, lung cancer might be rare.

Emphysema, like lung cancer, is attributed almost solely to smoking. Yet emphysema was rare until around 1960, although during the previous thirty years, smoking was even more prevalent than it was after the

1960s. However, between the end of World War II in 1946 and 1960, there was a tremendous growth in air-polluting industries. This transformed emphysema, which before that time was a rare disease, into one of epidemic proportions.

Anna and her husband, Olaf, who lived in Malmö, Sweden, moved to New York City when Olaf, who worked for a multinational paper company, was transferred to the New York office. Anna had not smoked as much as a single cigarette, but her lungs were so sensitive to the pollutants in the New York air that she had pneumonia six times during the twenty years she lived in New York City. Pneumonia, a bacterial or viral infection that inflames the alveolar sacs and causes them to fill with fluid, is a causative factor in emphysema. After her last bout of pneumonia, Anna developed emphysema. On the advice of her doctor she and Olaf left New York and settled permanently in their summer place in Nantucket, Massachusetts. Anna hasn't had pneumonia since.

Treatments That Detoxify the Lungs

Juiced vegetables, especially celery and dandelion juice, detoxify the lungs. The circulating blood carries this juice to the liver, which uses the alkaline minerals in the juice to neutralize metabolic wastes and heavy metals. The detoxified blood leaves the liver and eventually circulates in the lungs, where it neutralizes wastes trapped in the air sacs. Once cleared of this garbage, the inflamed air sacs and bronchioles have a chance to heal.

The chlorophyll molecules in vegetable juice, by rebuilding the hemoglobin molecules in the red blood cells, play a big part in enabling the lungs to take in more oxygen. This reconstruction is possible because of the similarity between the chlorophyll and hemoglobin molecules. Both contain a mineral— in chlorophyll it's magnesium; in hemoglobin, its iron—surrounded by carbon, nitrogen, and oxygen atoms in the same order. When any of the elements encircling the iron in hemoglobin are missing, the chlorophyll molecule in the juice replaces the missing atomic elements. Thus reconstituted, the positively charged iron in hemoglobin can once again exert its magnetism and pull out the negatively charged oxygen molecules in the air sacs of the lungs, with the result that more oxygen is absorbed into the blood.

Bio-Identical Hormones for the Lungs

Studies show that women who had their ovaries removed along with their uterus had a 17 percent greater chance of getting lung cancer than women who didn't have their ovaries removed along with their uterus. The researchers who conducted the study were perplexed at this finding. Two studies unraveled the mystery. They showed a relationship between increased levels of estrogen and a greater number of air sacs (alveoli) in the lungs. In one study, when the ovaries of immature female rats were removed, at reaching maturity they had fewer alveoli than the female rats that did not have their ovaries removed. In the other experiment the mature female rats that were given estrogen developed more alveoli than those female rats who didn't receive any estrogen.[9] Obviously when the ovaries are removed, less estrogen is produced, since the ovaries produce estrogen. These studies went a step further, proving that estrogen stimulates the growth of alveoli.

What isn't immediately evident is why a greater number of alveoli is a protection against lung cancer. But this can be easily deduced. Oxygen destroys cancer cells, so the more alveoli (air filters) in the lungs the greater the air (oxygen) intake, and thus the greater the chances that cancer cells in the lungs will be destroyed.

Estrogen's ability to increase the number of air sacs in the lungs is explained by one of its basic functions during pregnancy. Estrogen triggers the lungs into taking in extra oxygen, so the expectant mother can "breathe for two." It does so by destroying oxygen in the parts of the body other than the lungs. This signals the lungs that more oxygen is needed, so the lungs take in more oxygen and the fetus's oxygen needs are satisfied.

Given that both aging and menopause decrease the number of alveolar (air) sacs in the lungs and that estrogen can regenerate them, women and men who have emphysema or chronic obstructive pulmonary disease should take natural hormone supplements of estrogen. Menstruating women can take bio-identical hormone replacement therapy (BHRT). Pregnenolone serves the same function in men as BHRT does in women. Women who are still menstruating should take BHRT according to the rhythmic cycling of their menstrual month (see Chapter 16).

Improving Air Quality and Exercising the Lungs

You can improve the air in the home and workplace by using an air cleaner that produces negatively charged ions—or better yet, one that emits negative (alkaline) and positive (acidic) ions in the same ratio in which they occur in nature.

The volume of air we breathe into the lungs is also a factor in their health. Most of us don't breathe in enough air and, as a result, the lungs don't have the force to breathe out all the stale air lodged in the alveoli. This stale air takes up space, reducing the lungs' oxygen capacity. The easiest way to get rid of this stale air lodged in the lower lobes of the lungs is to become a deep breather.

The best exercise for strengthening the diaphragm and rib muscles so that the lungs can take in more oxygen and therefore have the force when exhaling to pull out the stale air, is by mimicking the panting of dogs—open your mouth, stick out your tongue, and breathe deeply. One individual who profited from this exercise was Jack Smith, a professional photographer. Jack developed emphysema at the age of seventy-three. He believes his exposure to asbestos was responsible. When he was twenty-seven, he took pictures of the interior of a naval ship while it was being sprayed with asbestos. He had forgotten about this until the diagnosis of emphysema jogged his memory. Jack's chiropractor recommended panting as a way to strengthen the alveoli, and Jack has performed this exercise for an hour each day ever since. He also bought an ionizing air cleaner for his apartment. A breathing test, taken a year after he began exercising his lungs and installed an air cleaner, showed that his breathing was almost normal (95 percent).

Too much exercise appears to have the same effect as emphysema in terms of preventing the lungs from breathing in enough oxygen. This is indicated by the results of the breathing tests taken by two groups of individuals, one comprising patients with emphysema and the other highly trained athletes. It was conducted by Carl Stough, a former opera singer who trains people with lung problems to breathe correctly. He writes in his book, *Dr. Breath*, that the results of the breathing tests of his emphysema clients were about the same as those of the Olympic sprinters in the control group![10]

SUGGESTIONS FOR EMPHYSEMA AND PNEUMONIA*

➤ **Dark green vegetables, including spinach, collard greens, chard, and kale.** The grain eater should eat them at least once a day, preferably raw; the meat eater, three times a week.

➤ **Raw vegetable juice.** Drink one pint of celery juice and three pints of a combination of carrot, spinach, and a small amount of watercress or parsley each day.

➤ **Ionizing air cleaner** (see Resources).

➤ **Castor oil packs.** Place on the liver for one hour a day for five to ten days (see Resources).

➤ **Vitamin A** (50,000 units/day). Before taking more than this amount, sometimes necessary in emphysema, consult your doctor.

➤ **Vitamin E** (800 to 1,600 units/day). It lessens the need for oxygen.

➤ **Vitamin C** (1,000 to 3,000 mg/day).

➤ **Chlorophyll.** Take two or more tablets three times a day (made by Standard Process).

➤ **Bio-identical hormone replacement therapy.** Use this in the form of a cream that is applied to the neck, inside the elbows, on the wrists, or anywhere else on the body where the blood vessels are close to the surface of the skin. Follow the directions on the label. Pregnenolone performs the same function for men as HRT does for women (see Chapter 16). For emphysema and chronic obstructive pulmonary disease.

➤ **Aangamik** (DMG) (250 mg three times a day). It is made by Food Science Labs.

➤ **Tea tree oil.** Taking one-quarter teaspoon three times daily for seven days is more effective than antibiotics in killing off the bacteria or viruses that cause pneumonia.

*Take as many of these nutrients as possible in the form of whole-food complexes. For dosage, follow the directions on the label.

CHAPTER 10

BONE HEALTH

B one degeneration has many causes. It can be brought about by an autoimmune disease, the lack of a key enzyme, a more pressing need for bone calcium elsewhere in the body, or a medication such as synthroid (used for underactive thyroid), which can lead to osteoporosis. But the greatest cause, and one that exacerbates existing degenerative bone disease, is the acid waste by-products of undigested food, heavy metals, and man-made chemicals. Circulating in the synovial fluid that surrounds the bones, it eats away at the bone mass.

Rheumatoid Arthritis and Osteoarthritis

Stephanie, age sixty, a children's dress designer, had very painful arthritis. Because of its severity, she was convinced that whatever imbalance in her body was responsible for the two staph infections and autoimmune disorder she had earlier in her life was also the cause of her arthritis. Her first staph infection, osteomyelitis, occurred when she was nine. It was in the bone marrow of her left femur (the bone that extends from the knee to the hip). The infection left her with minor bone damage and a slight limp. She caught the second staph infection when she was in her early thirties. While planting flowers in her garden, her index finger suddenly swelled up and turned bright red. Within a half hour the swelling and redness spread to the rest of her hand and began moving up her arm. The doctor came to the house and gave her antibiotic injections that killed off the infection and saved her life.

Staphylococcus bacteria in the soil where she was planting flowers had gotten into a joint in her finger, probably through a hangnail in the cuticle, and meeting no resistance from her immune system, had multiplied so fast that were it not for the antibiotics it would have overrun her entire body within an hour. Stephanie had no apparent aftereffects other than a deformed finger.

In her late thirties Stephanie became pregnant for the third time. During the second trimester of her pregnancy, her spleen, programmed to filter parasites from the blood and get rid of worn-out red blood cells, devoured the healthy red blood cells instead. Stephanie's red blood cell count fell drastically, her complexion turned a waxy yellow, and her gums were gray.

Stephanie had become the victim of an autoimmune disorder. The spleen, a fist-sized organ located behind the stomach, is an incredibly rich source of powerful immune cells called monocytes. The monocytes are programmed to filter dead red blood cells from the blood, along with other debris. Stephanie's monocytes were acting in reverse, destroying her healthy red blood cells (the spleen's monocytes also heal damaged hearts and other injured tissues). When cortisone injections failed to stop the irrational behavior of the monocytes, the surgeon in residence removed her spleen. The next instant Stephanie's face and gums turned a healthy pink. Four months after her operation, she delivered a healthy, full-term baby.

The removal of the spleen would seem to have put an end to Stephanie's autoimmune disorder, but at the age of fifty, her immune cells were once again attacking her body. She had developed rheumatoid arthritis. The arthritis started with the swelling of the joints of her fingers in both hands; the pain and swelling gradually extended to her wrists and then to her back. An MRI showed that the cartilage between three of her vertebrae had worn away. The pain she felt when she laid down was caused by nerves that were pinched by the vertebrae rubbing against each other. Stephanie underwent an operation to have the vertebrae fused. The operation relieved the pain somewhat, but she still had to wear a brace in bed to prevent severe back pain.

Medical scientists blame autoimmune reactions on overactive immune cells. Stephanie's staph infections, however, would seem to indicate that, at least in her younger years, her immune system was underactive. The osteomyelitis in her leg bone would never have developed if the immune system had sprung into action. And it didn't react at all to the rapidly multiplying bacteria that infected her finger while she was gardening. Furthermore, autoimmune diseases are much more prevalent among those with underactive immune systems. For example, rheumatoid arthritis is thirty times more common in individuals who have an immune deficiency disease called Bruton's syndrome than in individuals who don't have this syndrome.[1]

The Underlying Cause of Rheumatoid Arthritis and Osteoarthritis

The systemic nature of arthritis and other degenerative bone problems is a reminder that the circulating blood is the principal carrier of the toxic agents that cause disease. Australian scientists, researching the cause of arthritis, came up with part of the answer. They discovered that the thicker the blood the more likely the individual is to have osteoarthritis or rheumatoid arthritis.[2] They attribute the thickened blood to small blood clots in the capillaries that feed the bone joints. But then they veer off in the wrong direction by claiming that these small blood clots are wholly the result of high blood pressure and elevated cholesterol and triglycerides.

Holistic doctors, chiropractors, and naturopaths come closer to the answer when they point a finger at acid waste in the blood as the clotting agent that congeals the blood and leads to arthritis. But they take for granted that this acid waste is the naturally occurring by-product of metabolic function. This seems unlikely.

I've found that people with arthritis are exceptionally prone to food allergies. That explains why they have thick blood. Food allergens, contaminated by histamines, turn into acid waste particles. As they accumulate they stick together, and when this happens the blood thickens. The blood, congealed as a result of these wastes, is no longer diluted enough to transport nutrients and oxygen to the bones. As a result, the bone joints become malnourished and deteriorate. The "cement" (collagen) that holds the bone cells together is washed away by the surrounding waste-filled synovial fluid. The bones suffer another onslaught. To protect the alkaline pH of the blood, acid waste in the fluid surrounding the bone joints is encapsulated in calcium and deposited on the joints. Thus bone joints, already weakened from erosion and lack of nutrients, become arthritic.

In Stephanie's case, the food allergies and immune disorders she had starting at the age of nine laid the groundwork for her arthritis. Her food allergies were so severe that, for example, after eating only one egg, her chronic eczema spread over her entire body. Stephanie's severe allergies to foods explain her autoimmune disorder. Exposed to the corrosive acidity of the food allergens as it devours them, the immune cells become disoriented and confuse the body's tissues with that of invading pathogens.

Nutritional Treatment for Rheumatoid Arthritis and Osteoarthritis

Stephanie had been taking painkillers for several years, and while they brought her some relief, she was convinced they were responsible for the fact that her arthritis had gotten worse. Dr. Marc Darrow, a professor of medicine at UCLA with a practice in sports rehabilitation in Los Angeles, says the worsening of arthritis caused by anti-inflammatory drugs is not unusual because reducing inflammation in one area causes it to spread deeper into the tissues.[3] It would seem to me this happens because when inflammation is artificially eliminated by painkillers, the brain would become confused. It would wonder why, when the arthritic condition still exists, the inflammation—that is, the blood that transports additional nutrients and oxygen to the site of the injury—has suddenly disappeared. The brain tries to rectify the situation by getting the inflammation process going in another area as close to the original site of the arthritis as possible. As inflammation spreads and becomes chronic, it increases bone degeneration.

Darrow suggests using prolotherapy, which involves injecting a sugar water solution into a muscle or tendon where it is attached to the painful bone area. He says this causes blood to flow to the inflamed area. The blood stimulates the healing process.

Stephanie's first priority in trying to alleviate her arthritis was to detoxify the synovial fluid in the area around her calcified bone joints. The most effective detoxifier is freshly squeezed organic vegetable juice because it is made up of water, minerals, and protein, nearly the same composition as the synovial fluid. Stephanie drank three glasses of juice a day made from grapefruit, celery, spinach, and carrots. This combination provides a balance of alkaline and acid electrolytes (electrically charged minerals). The salicylic acid in the grapefruit helps dissolve calcium that encrusts the cartilage and bones and also removes toxins from the synovial (lymph) fluid; celery juice keeps the sludge in solution, and carrots and spinach facilitate its elimination from the colon.

Stephanie also stopped eating wheat because she was allergic to the gluten (wheat protein), a common allergy among those with arthritis. An effective supplement for arthritis sufferers, as well as for those with osteoporosis, is a fatty acid called cetyl myristate (see Resources). The chemist who discovered cetyl myristate got the idea it would be a cure for arthritis in humans because mice don't get arthritis, a fact he attributes to their having cetyl myristate, a chemical humans lack. Stephanie took the prescribed dosage of six tablets of cetyl myristate a day for six weeks, and by the end of the six-week period, she felt, she said, as though the arthritis had actually been lifted out of her body. Cetyl myristate also lowered her elevated blood pressure. The effectiveness of this fatty acid is confirmed in an independent study of the research and findings of Harry Diehl, an employee of the National Institutes of Health, who isolated the fatty acid from Swiss albino mice. Of the forty-eight participants in the study, all of whom had advanced rheumatoid arthritis, only two failed to show any improvement. This was attributed to their prolonged use of cortisone, which had severely damaged their livers.[4]

While the effectiveness of cetyl myristate is partly due to its lubrication of the bone joints and muscles, its greatest value lies in its ability to repair the cell membranes of the bone cells that have deteriorated due to insufficient amounts of fatty acid.

Bursitis and Gout

Emily, fifty-one, a Romanian by birth, immigrated to the United States with her husband and five-year-old daughter fifteen years ago and settled in New York City. Shortly after their arrival her husband developed a brain tumor and could no longer carry out his duties as the superintendent of an apartment building. Emily, despite her aches and pains from arthritis, "to put bread on the table," she said, took over her husband's job. Every morning she hauled plastic bags loaded with garbage from the basement up a flight of stairs and dragged them onto the curb; she swept the stairs and hallways and in the winter shoveled snow off the sidewalk in front of the building. Emily carried out these tasks despite wrists that were so stiff she couldn't turn a doorknob to open a door, throbbing pain in her toes, and heel spurs that made her feel, while walking, as if she couldn't carry the weight of her body. She also had bursitis in her shoulders and pains in most of her muscles.

Emily had probably inherited her bone problems from her father who had had gout. It caused him far more pain than Emily felt from all her bone problems put together. Gout develops from elevated levels of uric acid in the blood that are converted into sodium urate crystals and deposited in the toes, wrists, and earlobes. Joseph's gout started in the joints of his big toes and spread to the rest of his feet, inflaming and swelling the muscles. This eventually caused the muscles in his feet to degenerate. He became flatfooted and had to wear slippers even when he went out.

Emily used the best remedy possible for gout. She ate cherries, a treatment that Dr. Ludwig E. Blau tried on twelve individuals with gout, every one of whom experienced great relief. The remedy worked whether the cherries the subjects ate were canned or fresh, juiced or eaten whole.[5] Dr. Blau found that they were also effective in healing bursitis (calcification of the pockets of synovial fluid into which the bone joints in the shoulder fit).

Cherries remove the sodium urate crystals in and around the bone joints by dissolving them. Once dissolved, they are easily eliminated. How cherries dissolve the sodium urate crystals is another question, but it is likely that the acid in the cherries breaks them up, just as vinegar can break down the calcium deposits in arthritic bone joints. Emily got her quota of cherries in the form of a cherry liqueur that she made from an old Romanian folk recipe. She mixed sour cherries, unfiltered honey, blueberries, and vodka in a flat pan and left it in the sun for two weeks to ferment, then strained it. Drinking three cups of this highly nutritious, low-alcohol-content beverage daily for two to three weeks cured her gout as well as the bursitis in her shoulder.

J. P. Seegmitten in his book *Gout* writes that humans suffer from gout because they lack an enzyme called uricase that in animals converts uric acid into a more soluble substance.[6] In fact, humans don't need this enzyme. As long as normal levels of uric acid are maintained it's easily excreted from the urine. It is only when blood uric acid levels go so high that they endanger the stability of the blood's acid-alkaline balance (pH factor 7.4) that the excess uric acid is removed from the blood and deposited as far away from the major blood supplies as possible—in the toes, wrists, or earlobes.

Lowering Uric Acid Levels in the Blood

How can elevated uric acid blood levels be lowered? Because purine (a white crystalline compound) and nucleic acid break down into uric acid, doctors recommend that individuals with gout avoid eating foods with a high purine or nucleic acid content, such as liver, sweetbreads, game, herring, anchovies, lobster, crab, sardines, pork, and avocados. With the exception of pork, foods rich in purine and nucleic acid are, as a rule, not eaten often enough to cause gout.

The different types of arthritis Emily suffered from showed that she had a wide range of enzyme deficiencies. To remedy this, Emily took a supplement that contained enzymes that break down fat, protein, and starch. She also took ox bile powder to emulsify fat globules (see Resources). This enzymatic complex lessened the pains in her muscles, but it was the CoQ-10 she took that improved her digestion. Good digestion eliminates the acidic waste by-products of undigested food debris that end up in mineral deposits on bones, tendons, and muscles.

To reduce the size of the spurs in her heels, Emily underwent an ultrasound and paraffin wax treatment in a hospital. Her feet were dipped in hot wax ten times and then subjected to eight minutes of high-frequency sound waves. This alternative treatment, which is very popular with doctors in Germany, dissolved Emily's heel spurs. A few years later she took her husband to the hospital to have the same treatment, but the hospital had stopped the procedure, claiming that it didn't work. Emily said that no one had asked her whether the treatment helped her. She wonders if the medical staff at the hospital found it too much trouble to administer—or too controversial.

Emily used magnetic energy to take away the pain in her arthritic wrists. Attaching a magnetic pad to each wrist with a Velcro band, she wore them to bed at night. In a few days her wrists no longer ached.

Osteoporosis

My mother had osteoporosis. She wondered why she had excess calcium deposited on the surface of her bones where it wasn't supposed to be but didn't have enough calcium inside her bones where it should be. Of course, the calcium deposits on the surface of bone joints and vertebrae had once been part of her bone structure. She had suffered a loss of calcium either because there was a more pressing need for it elsewhere in her body or because acidic waste in the watery fluid surrounding the bones had dissolved some of the bone mass. The loss of bone mass in my mother's wrist bones when she was only thirty-five was so great that an x-ray showed them to be hollow.

Calcium is leached from the bones and absorbed by the blood when it is needed elsewhere in the body. Sufficient blood calcium is necessary for the nerves to perform such vital functions as controlling the heartbeat, regulating the secretion of hormones, and digesting and assimilating food. It also alkalinizes the nerves and blood when they are too acidic. In cases of hyperacidity, calcium is more important to the nerves and circulatory system than it is to the bones, so the body sacrifices bone mass to keep the pH of the blood balanced. Excessive acid in the arterial blood, a pH of 6.95, although not that much lower than the normal 7.4, can cause coma and death. To prevent this, alkaline-forming calcium combines with the excess acid and solidifies. It becomes calcium carbonate and is deposited on the bone joints and vertebrae.

The body reduces bone mass not only to obtain calcium but also to replenish its supply of energy. Enzymes split calcium molecules down the middle to release packets of energy, called adenosine triphosphate (ATP), tucked inside the calcium.

As hyperacidity in the blood and fluids surrounding the bones is the cause of all forms of bone degeneration, a diet that leaves behind as little acidic waste as possible is the first prerequisite (see Chapter 2). When acidity is reduced, it gives the joints a chance to heal. The second most important means of accomplishing this is to eat foods high in alkaline particles (electrons) and mucilage—partially cooked or raw potatoes, celery, and gelatin sprinkled on foods or in drinks. (For the best-quality gelatin, see Resources.) Gelatin also regenerates the bone because it contains a form of calcium that is more easily absorbed than any other.

Individuals with osteoporosis can take several measures to rebuild their bone mass so as to avoid the two major health problems that it causes: (1) fractures of the lower forearm and, in later life, of the hip, and (2) loss of height from curvature of the spine and legs. The mineral strontium is probably the most effective supplement for building bone mass in cases of osteoporosis. Strontium nourishes the cells whose function is to produce new bone cells and at the same time reduces the activity of the cells that dispose of worn-out bone cells.

If taken long enough strontium lactate—or in fact any form of strontium—can eliminate radioactive strontium-90 from the body. Strontium is structurally close to calcium as it is placed just below it on the periodic table. Its effectiveness depends on taking it on an empty stomach, a maximum of 1.7 g/day. Double the amount of calcium you take in relation to your strontium supplement. Boron as well as vitamin D help the body assimilate and utilize calcium. Magnesium also assists in the assimilation of bone calcium. But when calcium supplements don't relieve the pain of arthritis it can be because of a deficiency of boron, which prevents its absorption into the bones.

Besides the dietary measures already stated, alkaline water and far infrared (FIR) heat sleeping pads help stem bone loss by dissolving the acidic wastes in the fluids surrounding the bone joints and muscles.

Fibromyalgia

Shortly after Dorothy turned fifty-five, she retired as private secretary to the executive vice president of a pharmaceutical company. This was when she first felt a stabbing pain in her muscles. The pain gradually spread to all of her muscles and never let up. Around this time Dorothy's sleep patterns changed. She went from sleeping seven hours at night to sleeping most of the time. Besides muscle pain and fatigue, Dorothy experienced memory loss and such extreme dizziness that she often felt disoriented. Dorothy went out only once in the twelve months before she finally got control over her illness. A close friend drove her to Atlantic City on her birthday to gamble on the slot machines. The exertion intensified her pain for several days afterward. Dorothy went to a rheumatologist who diagnosed fibromyalgia and prescribed steroids.

Very little is known about fibromyalgia. However, a hypothesis is possible from the few facts that are understood. The debilitating pain of this disease begins in muscles located near the bone joints. This suggests that acidic wastes in the synovial fluid surrounding the bone joints cause inflammation and injury in fibromyalgia just as they do in arthritis. This, plus the fact that individuals with fibromyalgia experience chemical changes in the nervous system, suggests that nerves damaged by acid waste are the cause of fibromyalgia. The systemic nature of fibromyalgia is additional evidence that the nervous system is the injured organ in this disease, since the pain impulses travel along nerve pathways that extend into every part of the body.

It was hard to help Dorothy because of her unwillingness to make an effort to help herself. Being too ill to do much of anything, she needed a treatment that took no effort, so she slept on a far infrared sleeping pad. The heat produced by the electrical current goes through a layer of carbon inside the pad, creating the red spectrum of light that radiates deep inside the body and raises the internal temperature. This melts the pain-causing sharp acidic crystals, which are then eliminated through the kidneys, colon, or skin. After sleeping on an FIR pad for three months, Dorothy woke up one day to find that the pain in her body had vanished and the lymph nodes on the inside of her legs, under her arms, and on her neck were no longer sore to the touch. The explanation was obvious from the huge open sores all over her body. They were the means by which the toxic waste—dissolved by the far infrared heat energy and transported by the lymph system to the glands under the skin—were being eliminated from her body.

SUGGESTIONS FOR ARTHRITIS AND OTHER BONE DISEASES*

➤ **Progesterone.** Use a natural progesterone cream and follow directions on the label. Progesterone rebuilds bones, literally increasing the rate at which new bone is built. It is especially effective in osteoporosis. The decline in bone mass corresponds to a drop in progesterone during perimenopause.[7]

➤ **Calcium food complex.** Taking calcium without co-minerals can lead to osteoporosis.

➤ **Cetyl myristate.** Take six capsules daily for a maximum of six weeks. This is very effective for osteoarthitis and rheumatoid arthritis. It can also relieve the pain and soreness of fibromyalgia. This fatty acid works even better if it is taken with the other nutrients listed here.

➤ **Strontium** (200 to 400 mg/day to a maximum of 1.7 g/day). Strontium helps heal osteoporosis. Take on an empty stomach. Take calcium and strontium in the ratio of 2 to 1.

➤ **Gerovital** (200 mg/day). This medication is made up of procaine, which chemically is almost identical to the anesthetic dentists use. Gerovital can prevent arthritis.

➤ **Hyaluronic acid** (150 mg/day). See Resources.

➤ **Glucosamine sulfate** (1,000 mg/day). Glucosamine forms cushioning and lubricants between joints. Avoid chondroitin, as it can lead to cancer. Also, studies show it is not the chondroitin but the glucosamine sulfate that relieves arthritic pain.

➤ **Vitamin E** (800 to 1,600 units/day). Vitamin E prevents the destruction of fatty acids needed to build strong cell membranes in muscle and bone cells that keep out toxins.

➤ **A formula consisting of fish, primrose, and flaxseed oil.** This supplement relieves the swelling and pain of osteoarthritis. Don't take it without vitamin E, which prevents the toxic breakdown of these essential fatty acids.

continued

➤ **Omega-3, -6, and -9 fatty acids.** Nordic Natural makes a capsule that combines all three of these fatty acids. Take three capsules daily. Many people rave about the effectiveness of this formula in relieving arthritic pain.

➤ **B complex.** Take two to four capsules a day containing 100 mg each of vitamins B_1, B_2, B_3, and B_6 and at least 1,000 mcg of folic acid.

➤ **Vitamin B_{12} injections.** Dr. I. S. Klemes successfully treated shoulder bursitis with B_{12}. Since vitamin B is important in nerve function, B_{12} injections might also be effective in treating fibromyalgia.[8]

➤ **Thyroid extract.** Low thyroid function is one of the causes of arthritis. For natural thyroid supplements, see Chapter 5. If you have an underactive thyroid, before you begin taking thyroid medication, have your progesterone levels and parathyroid checked. Avoid synthetic thyroid medications if possible. Studies show they increase the risk of osteoporosis.

➤ **Calcium microcrystalline hydroxyapatite** (800 to 1,200 mg/day). Aside from gelatin, this is the most effective form of calcium because its tiny molecules can penetrate bone mass. Take it with its co-minerals and other factors because the intake of calcium without them can lead to osteoporosis.

➤ **Magnesium aspartate** (800 mg/day).

➤ **Raw egg yolk.** Eat one raw egg yolk daily, preferably fertilized eggs and from chickens that have been fed organically grown grains to avoid any chance of contracting salmonella. Raw eggs contain an abundance of pantothenic acid, which most individuals with arthritis are deficient in. When guinea pigs' diets were supplemented with egg yolk, they didn't develop allergy-induced arthritis. A good reason for pantothenic acid's effectiveness in preventing arthritis is its role in helping the body to dispose of acidic wastes.

*Take as many of these nutrients as possible in the form of whole-food complexes. For dosage, follow the directions on the label.

CHAPTER 11

EYE DISEASES

The eyes can't function without sunlight, for it's the sun's light rays that carry images through the eye to the screen in the back of the brain—which is where we see what is around us. If acid waste and free radicals have accumulated in the lens, clogged the eyes' drainage canal, or damaged the retina, the images we see become blurred. If wastes continue to accumulate, we can lose our sight altogether. Fortunately, the appropriate diet and nutrients can heal the eye by clearing out the calcified debris and rebalancing the eyes' acid-alkaline pH.

Cataracts

Frank is an example of someone who cured his eye problem by taking a vitamin and avoiding an allergy-causing food. A career army officer, he had been on combat duty in Korea. After the war he returned to the United States and was sent to an army base in Olympia, Washington. It was there that he became the victim of a freak accident. Waiting in the office at army headquarters to obtain some papers, he turned around to examine a partition that was being assembled as a room divider. Frank heard the sound of a drill, but it never occurred to him that the carpenter was drilling a hole on the other side of the partition he was looking at. What happened next took place in a fraction of a second. The drill broke through the composite board with such force that it went straight through Frank's eye all the way to the optic nerve and destroyed his sight in that eye.

The loss of his right eye didn't hold Frank back. Leaving the army a year after the accident, he received a B.A. in classical languages (Latin and Greek) and got a job teaching at a community college. There was just one downside to the loss of vision in one eye: He could no longer play tennis or Ping-Pong because depth perception is dependent on the blending of two separate images. He had lost the three-dimensional vision necessary for judging the distance between himself and the ball.

Frank's wife, Lorraine, worried that his good eye, doing the work of two eyes for more than forty years, had come under too much strain, and she urged Frank without success to take antioxidant vitamins. (The National Eye Institute and the Chinese Academy of Medicine in Beijing showed that in subjects between the ages of forty-five and seventy-four who took antioxidant vitamins the incidence of cataracts was reduced by 43 percent.[1]) Shortly after Frank celebrated his sixty-fifth birthday he began complaining that the red walls in the living room were so bright they hurt his eyes—although it was he who had insisted on painting the walls red. Now he wanted to repaint the walls blue, a color he had never liked.

When eyes become sensitive to a bright color, it is usually because particles have infiltrated the lens or cornea. The particles in the lens give the images a yellowish tint, and this changes the perception of colors. The colors with longer wavelengths such as red, orange, and yellow become too luminous, while those with shorter wavelengths such as blue and violet are by contrast restful. Although Frank didn't have the more common symptoms of a cataract such as seeing halos around images, fogginess, or loss of vision, the fact that he felt differently about colors meant that he was seeing them differently because his lens or cornea had become indistinct. The doctor examined his eye and found that in fact his lens was opaque in spots, a sign that a cataract was beginning to form.

How Cataracts Develop

The lens is a series of transparent layers of epithelial (skin) cells composed of approximately 60 percent water and 40 percent soluble materials, mostly protein. A lens develops a cataract for the same reason that arteries harden and bones become encrusted with calcium deposits: it has been injured by acidic waste. Calcium bonds with the waste to prevent the acid from making any more scratches or holes in the lens. The calcium deposited on the lens shows up as black spots, thus impeding vision.

Cataracts grow faster in the lens when energy production (respiration) slows. For when the lens is being covered over with a cataract, it can't absorb the nutrient it needs to make energy. That nutrient is vitamin B_2 (riboflavin). The lens relies on B_2, and to a lesser extent on vitamin C, to take the place of oxygen because it has no capillaries to supply it. (This makes sense, since capillaries in the lens would obstruct vision.) Dr. Sydenstricker of the University of Georgia and University of Georgia Hospital gave 15 mg of B_2 daily to forty-seven subjects. After nine months the cataracts in all forty-seven patients had disappeared.[2]

Another reason that the clouding of the lens increases when respiration (energy production) slows is that less carbon dioxide—the byproduct of respiration—is produced. When there isn't enough carbon dioxide to dispose of free radicals (free radicals are atoms that have lost an electron and go crazy in their effort to seize an electron from another atom) the lens clouds up even more. The importance of carbon dioxide in the prevention of cataracts is underscored by the fact that in Nepal, a country that is fifteen thousand feet above sea level, despite stronger sunlight at that altitude, cataracts are 2.7 times less common than in areas situated at lower altitudes.[3] This is because in mountainous areas where there is less oxygen, respiration is more efficient, so it gives off higher-than-average amounts of carbon dioxide. When healthy levels of carbon dioxide are maintained, the transparency of the lens is assured.

Frank wondered how he could have developed cataracts when he was such a careful eater. He shopped organic, ate vegetarian foods, the diet for his metabolic type, and drank a lot of carbonated bottled water. He found the answer to his question when he took his basal temperature. Over three days it averaged 97 degrees, an indication that his thyroid activity was depressed and therefore that his lens didn't have enough energy to burn up the waste products generated by its metabolic activities.

Since foods that the digestive tract can't break down properly can lower thyroid function, and since Frank was also experiencing severe stomach pains from gas, it seemed likely that a digestive problem had initiated his hypothyroid condition. Frank tested the foods he ate, one by one. When he eliminated whole-wheat bread his gas pains went away. This puzzled him because he could eat other wheat products such as couscous, wheat crackers, and whole-wheat pita bread without any ill effects. Bread, however, contains yeast, which none of the other wheat products in his diet did. By avoiding bread Frank also brought his temperature back up to 98.6 degrees. For his cataract-thickened lens to produce enough energy to eliminate his cataract, Frank took extra amounts of vitamin B_2. In six months his cataract disappeared. It had been broken up, dissolved, and eliminated, leaving Frank with a lens as clear as crystal.

SUGGESTIONS FOR CATARACTS*

➤ **Progesterone.** Topical natural progesterone relieves cataracts and other eye problems. Apply on the neck, on the wrists, or inside the elbows. Follow the directions on the label. (Use periodically.)

➤ **Thyroid supplements.** See Chapter 5 for more information.

➤ **Vitamin E** (400 to 800 units) **and coconut oil.** Taken together, these assist the thyroid supplements in normalizing thyroid function.

➤ **Riboflavin (B_2)** (15 to 50 mg/day). Along with vitamin C, riboflavin helps assure energy production in the lens.

➤ **Vitamin B complex.** Take a complex that contains 100 mg each of B_1, B_2, B_3, and B_6 three times a day.

➤ **Vitamin D** (1,000 units/day). Vitamin D assists in the absorption and utilization of calcium so that it doesn't become waste and harden the lens and cornea.

➤ **Vitamin A** (25,000 to 50,000 units/day).

➤ **Vitamin C** (1 g/day).

➤ **Avoid the use of microwave ovens.** Cataracts have been linked to microwave radiation.[4] Just as cooking an egg causes the white part of the egg to lose its transparency, so heat radiating from a microwave can elevate the temperature of the eye to the point where the lens gradually becomes opaque.

---

*Take as many of these nutrients as possible in the form of whole-food complexes. For dosage, follow the directions on the label.

Glaucoma

The diseases that afflict the eye are always related to congestion. In cataracts, particles and free radicals infiltrate the lens; in macular degeneration, the macula cells deteriorate and are replaced with alien molecules; and in glaucoma, the duct in which fluids flow to the outside of the eye becomes clogged. Wherever wastes in the eyes accumulate, the ability to see is jeopardized.

STEVE DEVELOPED GLAUCOMA, THE RESULT OF DEBRIS FROM AN INFECTION

Steve Abenega, age forty-three, a jazz musician living in New York, was born in Ghana, West Africa. He grew up along the Volta River where many of the inhabitants had developed glaucoma or cataracts, two diseases that were unknown until sometime after a dam on the Volta River was built in 1961.

After that, the joy of life began to ebb. First, the dam held back the nutrient-rich silt, so crops began to fail. Then the fish and crocodiles died, and the villagers were deprived of two foods they had relied on to supplement their protein requirements. Eventually the flow of the river stopped altogether. What was left was silt.

Steve and his friends played in their bare feet in the muddy silt. They paddled and splashed about in every patch of water they could find. Unbeknownst to them, buried in the silt in which they burrowed their feet were the larvae of the fluke and snail. These parasitic worms bore into the webbed skin between their toes. Once inside the bodies of these children, the larvae fulfilled their destiny. They swam through the blood upstream to the lungs, then to the liver, attracted by the density of its nutrients. The shistosomiasis worms (hatched from the larvae) pierce these organs, sucking the blood from them until they become like bleeding sponges. Those who are infected lose their strength and become apathetic. They also develop glaucoma or cataracts, in some cases both. The infection takes a long time to kill but is ultimately fatal.

continued

> Steve was saved by immigrating to the United States where he was given antibiotic treatments that cleared up his infection. But he suffered one aftereffect of the infection years later: glaucoma.
>
> His ophthalmologist wanted him to use eye drops, but Steve insisted on trying natural remedies first. He took vitamin C, bioflavonoids, and bilberry liquid extract. He also took the rest of the supplements on the "Suggestions for Glaucoma" list (see end of this section) for three months. After about six months, tests showed the pressure in his eye had dropped to 15, which was within the normal range.

How Glaucoma Develops

The interior of the eyeball is filled with a transparent jellylike fluid called vitreous humor. The pressure this thickened fluid exerts is what gives the eyeball its balloonlike contour. There is another, far smaller amount of fluid in the eyes that is more watery than vitreous humor, called aqueous humor. Located in a tiny chamber between the pupil and the lens, it does what the thick jellylike fluid can't do. It flows, and as it does so, it drops off nutrients and oxygen for the cornea and picks up waste products. The waste-filled watery fluid flows out of the chamber into a narrow canal and from there to the outside of the eye. This elimination process works well—unless the drainage canal becomes so clogged with waste that the fluid can't drain out of it. In a clogged canal or duct, this waste-filled fluid builds up and puts pressure on the vitreous humor in the interior of the eyeball. The vitreous humor, in turn, puts pressure on the retina in the back of the eye. If the pressure is great enough, it destroys the retina's nerve cells (the rods and cones) and causes blindness.

Eliminate Acidic Waste to Treat Glaucoma

The only way to save the eyes from going blind in glaucoma is to unclog the waste-filled duct so as to relieve the pressure on the retina. Massive doses of vitamin C can do this. Dr. Michele Virno, in an experimental research study, used 0.5 g of ascorbic acid for every 2.2 pounds of body weight of his human subjects. He published a paper in *Eye, Ear, Nose, and Throat Monthly* on the results.[5] According to the article, this massive amount of vitamin C dramatically reduced the intraocular pressure in glaucoma by converting toxic waste to a soluble form so that it could be carried away by the capillaries in the eye. Once the volume of waste in the eye fluids was reduced, the swelling of the drainage canal went down and the excess fluid drained out of the canal, thus eliminating the pressure. The problem is, how many people's gastrointestinal systems could handle that much vitamin C?

Where do the acid wastes come from that clog the drainage canal? The answer is in the blood vessels in the cornea. When these blood vessels develop leaks, waste debris flow out and enter the drainage canal, clogging it. The blood vessel walls, however, can be strengthened so that waste can't escape. The best formula for healing leaking blood vessels is the following: 1 g vitamin C and 1 g bioflavonoids three times a day, along with twenty drops of bilberry extract (for its bioflavonoid content) three times daily. Vitamin C and bioflavonoids are two of the most important building blocks of collagen, the "cement" that holds the cells together and so prevents seepage.

Pigment also helps heal glaucoma (as well as macular degeneration) because it absorbs the light-carrying images that enable us to see. Every time we open our eyes and absorb light rays, we lose some pigment. It must be replaced for our vision to remain intact. In glaucoma, eye pigment is destroyed by the buildup of pressure on the retina.

Even if we have healthy eyes, as we use them, pigment gets used up. The best way to take care of the eyes' pigment requirements is to eat a lot of vegetables and fruit that have the pigments the eyes need. Supplements are also useful in this regard. Lutein, a pigment similar to the color of the beta-carotene in carrots (called carotenoid pigment), prevents further deterioration to the cone and rod cells in the retina caused by pressure. It does so by replenishing a purple pigment called rhodopsin in the rod cells. Both lutein and rhodopsin, however, are diminished by the actions they take to preserve our eyesight and improve our vision. The retinene in rhodopsin, a yellow pigment that is a form of vitamin A, is lost every time rhodopsin splits into its component parts in order to help us see in the dark (rhodopsin is made of retinene and a protein called opsin). By the same token, a portion of the orange pigment lutein is lost every time it heals the rod cells in the retina.

Good night vision also depends on replacing pigment. Vitamin A maintains healthy eyes, but for glaucoma patients lutein is more effective. Besides bolstering the rod cells, lutein also improves the function of the cone cells on the periphery of the retina that help us see in bright light. Egg yolk is an excellent source of lutein.

SUGGESTIONS FOR GLAUCOMA*

➤ **Progesterone.** Glaucoma and other eye problems can be relieved quickly by applying topical (natural) progesterone wherever the blood vessels are close to the skin, such as the neck, the wrists, or inside the elbows.[6] (Use periodically.)

➤ **Vitamin complex.** Take 1 g vitamin C, 1 g bioflavonoids, and twenty drops of liquid bilberry extract three times a day.

➤ **Lutein** (20 mg/day).

➤ **Vitamin A** (25,000 to 50,000 units/day).

➤ **Copper and manganese** (3 mg/day).

➤ **Vitamin B₁** (100 mg/day).

➤ **Niacin** (100 mg twice daily).

➤ **Vitamin B complex.** Take two capsules a day.

➤ **Vitamin E** (400 to 1,600 units/day).

---

*Take as many as possible of these nutrients in the form of whole-food complexes. For dosage, follow the directions on the label.

Macular Degeneration

Macular degeneration is a loss of vision in the macula, the central portion of the retina in the back of the eye. The macula, a yellow-pigmented area, being in the middle of the retina, bears the brunt of the image-carrying light rays that are reflected on it. While the outer area of the retina picks up peripheral images, the macula absorbs the images we see when we look straight ahead. It is thanks to our central vision that we can calculate the distance between ourselves and whatever it is that we are looking at.

Because, as primates, depth perception is critical to our survival, nature strengthened our central vision by placing our eyes close together. However, we developed strong central vision at the expense of our peripheral vision. The macula, as the visual center of the eye and therefore the most active part, is for that reason more vulnerable to injury than the periphery of the retina or any other part of the eye. It's therefore not surprising that while in glaucoma the retina in the back of the eye is damaged from pressure due to the buildup of waste-filled fluid in the front of the eyeball, in macular degeneration, the macula triggers its own deterioration.

How Macular Degeneration Develops

In macular degeneration, vision becomes blurred because as normal cells and tissue in the macula in the back of the eye are lost or disintegrate, inappropriate tissue (blood vessels and alien molecules) move in to take their place. These abnormal and misplaced cells injure the macula by causing scar tissue to form. Scar tissue blurs vision because as light rays focus on the scarred macula they are bent out of shape. The blurring of the vision increases when the insulating layer between the macula and the blood vessels behind it breaks down. Leftover fluids from this breakdown leak into the macula and cause additional scarring. In the meantime, a yellowish substance called drusen fills in the space behind the macula where the insulating layer had once been. This blocks the macula from the blood vessels that supply it with oxygen and nutrients. When blockage has completely cut the macula off from the nutrients and oxygen it needs to function, the more serious form of macular degeneration, the "wet" version, sets in. In an effort to supply the deprived macula with oxygen, a blood vessel inducer called VEGF stimulates the growth of blood vessels inside the macula. Probably because they don't belong there these blood vessels rupture and bleed. Scars grow over the ruptured spots, and this increases the blurring of the macula's central vision, often making it impossible to see images.

In an effort to stem the loss of vision in macular degeneration, medical researchers have tried to prevent the growth of blood vessels in the macula by destroying VEGF, the blood vessel inducer. Why don't these researchers instead try to find a way to detoxify the area behind the macula so that blood vessels will once again grow there? If the blood vessels are growing where they are supposed to grow, they will provide nourishment for the macula, possibly restoring the macula's central vision. Preventing macular degeneration from getting worse depends on reducing toxic waste levels in the eye so as to clear away the waste material that sets up a barricade between the macula and the oxygen-carrying blood vessels behind it.

Treating Macular Degeneration

Besides a junk-free, metabolically appropriate diet, the most important single nutrient in treating macular degeneration is zinc. The enzymes whose function is neutralizing aberrant chemicals in the macula can't do so without zinc as a coenzyme. Dr. David A. Newsome of the Louisiana State Eye Center in New Orleans conducted a research experiment in which he gave half of the 151 subjects, who all had macular degeneration, 100 mg of zinc twice a day, while the other half received a placebo.[7] Examined between one and two years after the experiment began, the subjects who took the zinc were found to have better vision than the ones who received a placebo.

Another way of assuring that the macula gets a normal supply of oxygen is by taking antioxidant supplements such as vitamins E and C and selenium. They make more oxygen available by preventing its breakdown, and vitamins E and C dispose of waste by absorbing the alien molecules that have invaded the macula. Oxygenating magnetic or far infrared pads placed over the eyes at night during sleep have the advantage of targeting the area where oxygen is needed most. The fact that a sufficient supply of oxygen helps ensure the production of normal energy levels in the rod cells in the macula is particularly important in light of the fact that 10 percent of those with macular degeneration go on to develop the more serious wet form of the disease.

Could a deficiency of yellow pigment (retinene) in the photosensitive rod cells in the macula be one cause of macular degeneration? The answer is yes, judging from a recent research study.[8] This study shows that people who eat one carrot daily—or any other beta-carotene-rich vegetable, such as spinach—reduce their chances of developing macular degeneration by 40 percent as compared to those who eat such foods less than once a week. Blueberries have also been shown to slow the loss of vision in macular degeneration, probably for the same reason that carrots do: the pigment in the blueberries is absorbed by the rod cells, enabling them to soak up the light rays reflected on the retina. When individuals don't have enough pigment to absorb all the light rays that fall within the range of the macula, it's difficult for their eyes to adjust to extremes of light. Either bright light hurts their eyes or they have trouble seeing in the dark.

Toxins such as tar and nicotine in cigarette smoke have ultimately the same effect on the rod cells in the eyes as too little pigment or too much acidic waste. The individual who smokes one or more packs of cigarettes a day is 2.4 times more likely to develop macular degeneration than someone who has never smoked. Nicotine destroys oxygen, which causes the cells to become inflamed and deteriorate. Unfortunately, longtime smokers who give up smoking seldom reduce their chances of getting macular degeneration. The tar and the nicotine in the cigarettes have already damaged the macula.

The breakdown of its communication system also helps destroy vision in the macula. This system, embracing all the cells in the macula, works only as long as the ions (electrically charged atoms) "jump" from one macula cell to the next, leaving behind an electrical charge. When the macula cells lose the ability to vibrate, it's a sign that this "electrical" network is broken and the cells have lost touch with each other.

Nutritional supplements can help repair the macula cells, but they can't recharge the cells' batteries. There is a device, however, called Frequency Specific Microcurrent (FSM), that can. It delivers an electrical current to the injured eye cells by way of tiny electrodes attached to acupuncture sites near the eye. These electrodes vibrate at the same frequency as the injured cells. The tissues (the muscles, tendons, bone) and conditions (scar tissue, inflammation, enzyme- or mineral-starved tissue) each have their own frequency, and the device's microcurrent frequency can be adjusted to match them.

The electrical currents emitted by the FSM, which are the same frequency as the degenerated macular cells, have been shown to increase the production of energy in these damaged cells by 500 percent. With this expanded energy, the injured macular cells can neutralize intracellular acid waste and then regenerate. Robert J. Rowen, M.D., sums up what the FSM does: "It restores the natural flow of electrical energy in the eyes of people with macular degeneration."[9] It is not surprising that this device has been given general approval by the FDA, because the electric current it generates is so tiny it is measured in millionths of an amp. (See Resources for more information on this device.)

SUGGESTIONS FOR MACULAR DEGENERATION*

➤ **Zinc** (50 mg/day).
➤ **Blueberries.** These berries contain bioflavonoids that build cell membranes and supply the retina with pigment.
➤ **Vitamin E** (400 to 800 units/day). Take with selenium.
➤ **Vitamin A** (25,000 to 50,000 units/day).
➤ **Vitamin D** (1,000 to 2,000 units/day).
➤ **Magnetic pad placed over the eyes** (see Resources).
➤ **Vitamin C** (1,000 mg/day).
➤ **Taurine, lutein, and zeaxanthin.** These are major constituents of the pigments in the retina. For dosage, follow the directions on the label.

---

*Take as many of these nutrients as possible in the form of whole-food complexes. For dosage, follow the directions on the label.

CHAPTER 12

DIABETES

M ore than 90 percent of adult Pima Indians living in the Sonora
desert in Arizona today are morbidly obese and diabetic by the
time they are in their thirties. This wasn't always the case. Before the
arrival of the European settlers, these indigenous peoples didn't have a
weight problem and diabetes was rare. Their good health was based on
a healthy diet and the fact that their digestive metabolism had adapted
to the weather pattern in the Sonora desert—six months of rain followed by a six-month period of drought. During the rainy season they
cultivated crops and gorged on tepary beans, melons, squash, and corn.
Because for the next six months there would be no rain and food would
be scarce, their bodies converted the food they ate during the wet season into fat and stored it in the body's fat cells. When the rain stopped
and the landscape reverted to desert, they lived off their body fat. The
hunger for food during this period of dryness almost disappeared.

Constantly craving food when it was available and losing the craving
for food when it was scarce meant that once food was accessible all year
long, the craving aspect of the appestat mechanism would become permanent. So when corner grocery stores opened in the Sonora desert, the
cycle of feast and famine ended and was replaced by nonstop gluttony.[1]

How Diabetes Develops

If gorging on excessive quantities of food and a diet of processed foods
and refined sugar and flour causes diabetes (high blood sugar), those

whose food intake is moderate—who eat a limited amount of sweets but lots of foods containing nutrient-rich fiber—are not likely to have high blood sugar and suffer from diabetes. In fiber-rich foods, the fibers are broken down gradually, with the result that glucose is released in a slow, steady stream. This makes it possible for all the blood sugar to be absorbed into the cells and utilized to generate energy. On the other hand, a diet high in refined sugar and flour is converted into glucose so quickly that blood sugar becomes elevated, and if there is not enough insulin to transport it to the cells, blood sugar levels remain high.

In those who have efficient insulin-producing beta cells, the excess glucose that can't be absorbed by the cells is carried by the blood to the liver where it is converted into glycogen (starch). When it is needed, it is converted back into sugar and gradually siphoned into the blood.

But when the liver is so overloaded with sugar that it can no longer absorb it, the pancreas releases additional insulin, which transports the excess blood sugar to cells that synthesize it into fat. When neither of these alternatives is an option, blood sugar levels, being chronically high, spill over into the urine. When tests reveal sugar in the urine, the diagnosis is diabetes.

Type 2 Diabetes

Type 2 diabetes, formerly referred to as adult-onset diabetes because it usually affected individuals past fifty, is the most common form of the disease—90 percent of those with diabetes have the type 2 form.[2] In recent years, however, it has become a disease of young adults and even children as well as the middle-aged and older segments of the population. Young adults are harder hit by type 2 diabetes than preceding generations because the processed foods they eat were less common when older generations were growing up.

Betty, age fifty, who worked as a secretary for an insurance company, had pain, numbness, and tingling in her wrists, the symptoms of carpal tunnel syndrome, a health problem associated with diabetes. John Ellis, M.D., wrote that 27.2 percent of the carpal tunnel patients of a Dr. George Phalen either had diabetes or had a family history of it. Two years later Betty developed insulin-resistant type 2 diabetes. Although insulin-resistant patients produce enough insulin, the insulin doesn't lower their blood sugar because it is unable to transfer sugar molecules from the blood into the cells. Betty had trouble believing that carpal tunnel and diabetes were related, since the conditions that trigger them are entirely different. The inflamed tissues in carpal tunnel, a narrow passageway in the wrist, are associated with repetitive wrist motions such as those involved in typing, while diabetes is caused by eating too much sugar or refined flour and sugar products. Betty spent her entire workday transcribing tapes onto a computer. She also consumed plenty of sugar. The company she worked for kept its underpaid employees happy by having the best bakery in New York deliver a cake, consisting mostly of icing, to the office every afternoon. Betty had been eating two hefty slices of this cake every day for the past twenty years, the period of time she had been working for the firm.

The condition that diabetes and carpal tunnel syndrome have in common is a deficiency of vitamin B_6. Dr. Kilmer McCully's research into homocysteine as a possible cause of atherosclerosis laid the groundwork for Dr. Ellis's discovery of the role it plays in diabetes and carpal tunnel.[3] (For more on atherosclerosis, see Chapter 6.) McCully proved that excess homocysteine (an amino acid used in the repair and generation of new cells), caused by a deficiency of vitamin B_6 and the enzyme that activates it, triggers hardening of the arteries. (Some studies, showing no relationship between elevated homocysteine levels and heart disease, have not confirmed McCully's findings.) The supplements McCully gave his research subjects, namely, vitamins B_6, B_{12}, and folic acid, made their arteries more flexible and acted as heart attack preventatives. Ellis, a medical doctor and researcher, noting that his patients with diabetes and carpal tunnel syndrome, like McCully's heart patients, suffered from a vitamin B_6 deficiency, concluded that they also had elevated homocysteine levels. He prescribed 100 to 200 mg/day of B_6 for these patients. The treatment alleviated both the carpal tunnel syndrome and the diabetes, indicating that excess homocysteine not only injures the arteries but is also a contributing factor in both diseases. On the basis of this research I recommended that Betty take 150 mg/day of B_6. Before long her blood sugar normalized and the pain and tingling in her wrists lessened.

It's most likely that in carpal tunnel syndrome, excess homocysteine accumulates in the ligaments in the carpal tunnel area of the wrist and causes them to become inflamed. Homocysteine's role in diabetes isn't quite so obvious. But given the high blood glucose levels in diabetics who have normal insulin levels, a logical explanation is that glucose (transported by insulin) can no longer penetrate the cells because the membranes of the cells have been hardened by homocysteine wastes.

Symptoms and Health Consequences of Diabetes

Once some of the glucose in the blood flows into the urine, the body's water reserves increase the volume of urine so that the urine is diluted enough to dissolve the sugar. So much of the body's water supply is used up in this way that the diabetic patient develops excessive thirst. Other symptoms of diabetes are weight loss, extreme hunger, and fatigue. These symptoms are caused by reduced energy production due to the fact that sugar is not being transported into the cells and used to manufacture energy.

The diabetic's whole body takes a toll when blood sugar becomes chronically high. For as the diabetics' sugar-saturated blood circulates through the organs, the sharp, pointed acid particles of sugar injure organ tissues. They become inflamed and harden. The hardening causes a loss of permeability making it difficult for the cells to absorb nutrients and oxygen. When the cells become so stiff and hard that they can no longer absorb any nourishment or air, they die. The eyesight is often the first to go. The microscopic blood vessels in the retina in the back of the eye harden, causing blurred vision and, if the diabetic lives long enough, blindness. The National Society for the Prevention of Blindness has found that 50 percent of those who have had diabetes for twenty years develop neuropathy (nerve damage) of the eyes, while 90 percent who have had diabetes for thirty years develop it. Studies by this agency also show that diabetes is the leading cause of blindness.

Elevated blood sugar also causes cataracts, breaks down the retina, hardens the arteries and heart tissue, and destroys nerves. Other parts of the body that are damaged in diabetics are the extremities, particularly the feet and legs. This begins when cuts, scratches, and rashes take longer to heal than they should. Eventually abrasions stop healing altogether. The cells, choked with metabolic wastes and starved for nutrients, die out, causing the flesh to rot and become gangrenous. Amputation prevents death—until the gangrene spreads to vital organs.

Treating Diabetes

The single most effective treatment for both type 1 and type 2 diabetes is lipoic acid.[4] The most easily absorbed form, alpha lipoic acid, eliminates the major symptom of diabetes, high blood sugar, by converting the excess glucose into energy. This helps solve other medical problems associated with diabetes, especially in the case of insulin-dependent diabetes. When lipoic acid normalizes blood sugar, the latter no longer injures the eyes, nerves, cardiovascular system, or extremities of the body. According to Dr. Hans Tritschler's clinical studies in Munich, Germany, lipoic acid, by lowering blood sugar levels, regenerates nerve damage caused when blood sugar levels spike.[5]

Lipoic acid can reduce elevated blood sugar levels by triggering the movement of the glucose transporters, a component involved in the blood sugar's entry into the cells. Like vehicles that leave the garage where they are stored and go wherever they are needed, glucose transporters, when blood sugar levels are normal, move from the interior of the cell to the cellular membrane, pick up glucose, and transport it into the cell.

But when blood sugar levels are too high, glucose transporters no longer act as blood sugar carriers. However, with the help of lipoic acid, they are able once again to convey the sugar molecules in the blood across the cellular membrane into the cell. Since lipoic acid contributes to the production of energy (which is packaged in units called ATP), it is not surprising that Dr. M. Khamaigi's group at the University of Negev in Israel[6] was able to prove that with increased levels of glucose inside the cells, thanks to lipoic acid, energy production increases.

FREE RADICALS: THE BODY'S ROGUE CELLS

Free radicals, a by-product of oxidation (the burning of glucose for energy), are missing an electron. This destabilizes them so that they go on a rampage, seeking to "steal" electrons from other molecules to replace the electrons they no longer have. Antioxidants like vitamins A, C, and E, beta-carotene, melatonin, and especially lipoic acid give up electrons to these free radicals gone berserk and, in doing so, stabilize them so they do no further damage.

Type 1 Diabetes and Insulin Transplant Operations

More than a decade ago, there was great excitement in the press over reports of the success of insulin transplant operations. Taken from the pancreases of deceased donors, insulin-producing cells were transplanted into the liver of patients with severe type 1 diabetes. The eight patients who had this procedure done two to fourteen months before it was publicized in the press no longer had any symptoms of the disease and so did not need insulin injections.

The skeptics (including myself) turned out to be right. The transplanted cells did not stand the test of time. A study that came out in 2006 in the *New England Journal of Medicine* found that the transplanted insulin-producing cells had freed patients with the severe form of diabetes from insulin injections for only two years. At the end of that time, 80 percent of the patients had gone back to intravenous insulin.[7]

The fact is that type 2 diabetes and even type 1 diabetes have been cured by using a far less traumatic procedure than surgery—and that is diet. This is the avenue therefore that even type 1 diabetics should explore—while they continue taking insulin—before consigning themselves to a lifetime of insulin injections.

HOW ALBERT CURED HIS INSULIN-DEPENDENT (TYPE 1) DIABETES

Albert had had a heart attack many years before he became diabetic. Like most individuals with emotional problems, Albert's temperament drove his behavior. On the day he closed up his ironwork shop for the last time, he became so angry that he smashed all the machinery and furniture in the shop. That night he had a heart attack.

Albert recuperated quickly, however, and remained in good health for twenty-eight years, until at the age of sixty-eight, he developed the symptoms of diabetes: trembling, dizziness, excessive thirst, and extreme hunger. Despite eating all the time, he lost weight. Diagnosed with insulin-dependent (type 1) diabetes, he had also developed elevated triglycerides and cholesterol.

Albert had always had a fear of needles, so he went through the tortures of the damned every time he injected himself with insulin. Out of desperation, an idea struck him that he could control his diabetes if he ate the right foods. When he had threatened to stop the insulin and the doctor warned him this was a death sentence, he agreed to stay on the insulin while he followed a diet that he hoped would cure his insulin problem.

He took the niacin test, found out that he was a grain eater, and went on the grain eater's diet with the objective of lowering his excessive blood sugar. Henceforth he avoided refined carbohydrates and ate vegetables in place of the large quantities of fruit he had eaten before. This reduced his overload of blood sugar.

Most seriously ill people who go on a diet to improve their health go off it once their fear of dying subsides. But Albert stuck to his diet. After he had been on the grain eater's diet for diabetics for three months, his elevated triglycerides and cholesterol dropped, and the Clinistix strip he waved in his stream of urine no longer turned red. This was a sign that his urine was sugar free. The doctor gradually cut down on his insulin, from 45 units to 30 and then to 15.

Six weeks later, Albert went off insulin altogether. A year after he had begun injecting himself with insulin, he was able to control his diabetes entirely through diet. Albert may very well be one of the few people with type 1 diabetes who had cured himself through diet, but that his case is not an anomaly is proven by my knowledge of four other people with type 1 diabetes who were also successful in using diet to wean themselves off insulin.

Type 1 Diabetes Prevention in Children

If you are planning to get pregnant, are already pregnant, or have given birth, the following information is worth taking seriously. A study, published in 2001 in the British medical journal *Lancet*, of ten thousand subjects revealed that those children in the study who were given vitamin D for one year after birth had 80 percent less type 1 diabetes over the next thirty-one years than those who received no supplements.[8] Other studies show that taking cod liver oil regularly also reduces the risk of type 1 diabetes in children.

SUGGESTIONS FOR DIABETES*

➤ **Cod liver oil.** For type 1 diabetes prevention in children, two tablespoons a day of cod liver oil for prospective parents and for their babies. (Cod liver oil can be purchased at a health-food store.) Keep children on cod liver oil for at least the first five or six years of their lives.

➤ **Bitter-tasting vegetables:** endive, spinach, beet greens, bitter melon (available at Chinese markets), and kerala, the Indian version of bitter melon (available at Indian markets). These foods lower blood sugar.

➤ **Vegetable juice.** The alkalizing effect of vegetables has been known to reverse type 1 diabetes if it hasn't become chronic.

➤ **Vitamin E** (400 to 800 units/day). Vitamin E helps normalize thyroid function and improve the sex drive in male diabetics.

➤ **Thyroid supplements** (see Chapter 5).

➤ **Alpha lipoic acid** (200 to 600 mg/day). For diabetic neuropathy, 600 mg/day improves nerve function.

➤ **Evening primrose oil** (360 to 480 mg/day). This strengthens nerve function, as do flaxseed and fish oil.

➤ **Vitamins B$_{12}$** (1,000 mcg/day), B$_1$ (100 mg/day), B$_6$ (100 to 200 mg/day), **and folic acid** (800 mcg/day). These B vitamins help reduce excess levels of homocysteine, which in turn reduces hardening of the veins and arteries in the liver and pancreas of diabetics.

➤ **Chromium picolinate** (400 to 600 mcg/day). This helps insulin transport glucose into the cells.

➤ **Gelatin.** Start with one-half to one ounce in liquid or sprinkled on food (see Resources). The mucilage in gelatin stabilizes blood glucose.

---

*Take as many as possible of these nutrients in the form of whole-food complexes. Follow the directions on the label for dosage.

CHAPTER 13

INSOMNIA

If you have trouble falling asleep at night, the most likely cause is acid indigestion from food you ate during the day. That's why the most important time of the day to eat foods compatible with your metabolic type is in the evening. People who eat the wrong foods for dinner or right before they go to bed often feel restless. This is a little recognized symptom of indigestion that can prevent sleep. Other causes of insomnia may result from stimulants such as caffeine, nicotine, and salt.

The individual who goes to sleep easily but wakes up later at night and can't go back to sleep is often addicted to eating large quantities of sugary foods, causing a rush of insulin that lowers the blood sugar too drastically. The result is hypoglycemia (low blood sugar), which brings on dizziness, depression, nervousness, indigestion, muscle pains, worrying, and so on—all of which can cause insomnia.

Hypoglycemia can also slow thyroid function, which triggers wakefulness. I have a meat-eating metabolism and a slightly underactive thyroid and probably a mild case of hypoglycemia, so when I wake up at 5:00 in the morning and can't get back to sleep I eat a few slices of red meat—a food appropriate to my meat-eating metabolism. It puts me to sleep immediately. My husband also used to wake up at 5:00 in the morning because of an underactive thyroid. Once he began taking thyroid supplements, he was able to sleep through the night.

A Brief History of Sleep

While the various systems inside our bodies speed up and slow down in tandem with night and day, we have not synchronized our waking and sleeping patterns with any such exactness. In the seventeenth century, before the electric lightbulb was invented, and even before the use of oil and gas lamps, people went through alternating periods of sleep and wakefulness at night. While they went to sleep as soon as it got dark, they awakened periodically during the night. During the time they were awake they meditated, chatted with their bedfellows—since before the twentieth century families typically shared the same bed—visited neighbors, or worked by candlelight.[1] This was such a widely established pattern that people commonly referred to their first and second sleep. Thomas A. Wehr of the National Institute of Mental Health did a research study that showed that when subjects were deprived of artificial light they reverted to the preindustrial sleeping mode and were asleep and awake in turns during the night. Wehr believes this adaptation occurred because, without artificial light, prolactin hormone levels, which bring about "a state of quiet restfulness," were raised.

Thus even when the only means of lighting up the darkness was the candle, people were defying the pineal gland's orders—delivered by its messenger melatonin—to sleep while it was dark and not wake up until the first sign of sunlight. People viewed wakefulness at night as entirely natural. Roger Williams, professor of biochemistry at the University of Texas in the mid- to late twentieth century, told me that waking up at night shouldn't be labeled insomnia or considered unhealthy if sleep that was lost at night was made up during the day.

In Spain and Greece people commonly sleep two hours every afternoon and then stay up very late at night. When I was staying at a hotel in Madrid, I was awakened at 4:00 A.M. by people talking on the street. Yet in the daytime the streets in this major metropolitan city were empty. In these Mediterranean countries people don't observe the day-night cycle because when the sun is directly overhead the heat is so intense it saps the body of energy, making it almost impossible to work. For the same reason, Middle Easterners who live in the desert turn the daily cycle of light and darkness upside down by sleeping in the daytime and at night searching for oases of grass and water to feed their camels and sheep.

Benefits of Dreaming

There are two kinds of sleep: the sleep when we don't dream, called orthodox sleep, which gets progressively deeper in four successive stages; and a shorter period of sleep when we dream. Dream sleep is called rapid eye movement, or REM, because while we dream the eyeballs move rapidly. Some researchers think these two kinds of sleep alternate in cycles throughout the night and that three-quarters of the time we experience orthodox sleep and the other quarter REM sleep. Dreams are most vivid the last two hours of an eight-hour period of sleep.

Medical science has different opinions as to whether there are biological or mental benefits to dreaming. The fact that dreaming is almost universal suggests it plays an important role in our health. There are indications that not having dreams is unnatural. For example, in a mental illness such as schizophrenia, as symptoms worsen, the victim dreams less and less and finally stops dreaming altogether. Also, people who regularly dream often become disoriented and anxious when a medication they are taking prevents them from dreaming. The fears, resentments, and anxieties we experience during our waking hours are often played out in our dreams, which is probably why nightmares are so common. It is possible that bad dreams, by giving us a chance to get the negative feelings "out of our system," lower stress hormone levels that rise when we become anxious or depressed.

A study consisting of seventy-seven volunteers reveals that dreaming can improve cognitive thinking.[2] The subjects were given a word association test and then underwent three different conditions: one group spent a day without a nap, another group napped without REM (dream) sleep, and the third group dreamed while napping. Spending a day without sleep and napping without dreaming both led to slightly better performances when the subjects were retested. But the group who dreamed while they napped had a 40 percent higher score than the other two groups.

Benefits of Sleeping in Complete Darkness

Many indigenous people don't have windows or any other opening in the walls of their huts because they believe in sleeping in complete darkness.[3] This makes sense in light of what we know about the hormone melatonin. The flow of melatonin, which puts us to sleep, needs complete darkness for optimal function. The slightest amount of light reduces melatonin production. Dr. David Blask, an oncologist at Bassett Research Institute in Cooperstown, New York, lowered the melatonin production of rats by exposing them to light while they slept. He then transplanted malignant tumors into the bodies of two groups of rats: one group had been exposed to dim light while asleep and the other group slept in total darkness. The tumors in the rats exposed to faint light grew much faster than those in the rats that slept in total darkness. This is probably because melatonin suppresses estrogen production and estrogen has been linked to cancer. Studies of blind women in Sweden and Finland support Blask's experiment. Those women who couldn't perceive any light at night had 60 percent less breast cancer. With the increase in the perception of light by some of the blind women, their rate of breast cancer rose. The decrease in cancer in those women who could perceive no light in the darkness proves that the less light exposure while sleeping, the greater the melatonin production, which automatically lowers estrogen. How dark then should we make the rooms in which we sleep? Since tests have shown that the eyes respond to moonlight and light from the street that filters through a window, either windows should be covered with opaque blinds that let no light through or eye masks should be worn.

The quality of sleep, however, depends not only on blocking out all light from the eyes but also on absorbing light through the eyes while we are awake. In fact, strong light works better than any natural supplement or drug medication in putting people to sleep at night. Those who develop SAD (seasonal affective disorder) from lack of sunlight during the winter and who use high-intensity, full-spectrum fluorescent lights to alleviate their symptoms of depression discover that they also sleep better.

How could exposure to intense natural or artificial light improve the quality of sleep when the act of sleeping is triggered by darkness? According to Dr. Dale Edgar, during the day, the more light we are exposed to, the more pressure builds up to sleep. Light, then, is not only a wake-up call; it also sets in motion the desire to sleep, and it does so by keeping our internal clock wound. Spending a block of time outside every day helps us sleep for another reason: it helps normalize thyroid function.[4] This is important because falling into a state of hypothyroidism makes normal sleep next to impossible.

How Much Sleep Is Enough?

The amount of sleep individuals need varies. Some people, mostly men, don't need more than five hours of sleep a night. Others need as much as twelve hours to be productive and alert during the day. While in college I read about a research study on sleeping patterns and their effects on longevity in a journal whose name I've long since forgotten. The study made an indelible impression because researchers tracked the sleep habits and life spans of sixty thousand subjects. It showed that those who slept seven hours nightly lived the longest. Eight-hour sleepers lived almost as long. However, sleeping even one hour over the standard eight hours sharply curtailed longevity, whereas individuals who slept less than seven hours, even those who slept only four or five hours a night, lived almost as long as the seven-hour sleepers. Seven hours of sleep may very well be most conducive to health and longevity, but if you feel rested and alert only by sleeping longer, curtailing your sleeping hours because it might extend your life for a few months would be counterproductive.

How to Treat Insomnia

The most effective antidote for insomnia, of course, is a healthy, metabolically appropriate diet. When digestion is complete we have no symptoms of indigestion, and when we feel well, we fall into a state of calm that is conducive to sleep.

Avoiding eating before you go to sleep is helpful because digestive problems arising from the evening meal are more likely to be resolved by the time you rest your head on the pillow. There are people, however, who insist they can't go to sleep on an empty stomach. Often the problem is not hunger or a feeling of emptiness in the stomach as they think it is but acidity. This is usually the result of acidic waste from undigested food debris. But it can also be caused by abnormally large quantities of stomach acid—an unbalanced digestive metabolism.

How this problem is resolved depends on your metabolic type. I learned recently from an Indian naturopathic physician that in India lime juice in water is recommended for acid indigestion. This makes sense because almost all Indians have grain-eating metabolisms and the high acid content of lime juice would help overcome the grain eater's natural deficiency in stomach acids. My experience confirms the value of this remedy as a sleeping potion. I've recommended it to a number of grain eaters who tell me it is an excellent sleep remedy. I'm sure it works by curing indigestion. Lime juice solves two problems at the same time. In normalizing inadequate acid levels in the stomach, any remaining undigested food in the stomach is broken down, a condition that induces sleep.

Meat eaters who have insomnia need an alkaline rather than an acidic remedy like lime juice because of their overload of digestive acid. Raw potatoes work very well for meat eaters. Chewing the crunchy potatoes to a pulp creates starchy alkaline juice that neutralizes the excess acid, whether it's an overload of hydrochloric (digestive) acid or acidic waste from incomplete digestion. Sleep is rarely a problem for the meat eater who uses the raw potato digestive remedy. An ice pack on the stomach of grain eaters and meat eaters who are in the throes of indigestion, along with the natural food remedy appropriate to the metabolism, is an effective means of bringing on sleep.

While the wrong foods are the prime cause of sleeplessness, there is another reason for insomnia related to the sleeping-waking timetable in our bodies. The gland that controls this biological clock is the pineal, located in the middle of the brain. It is thanks to the pineal gland that we have an internal link to the environment outside the body. The pineal synchronizes our lives with the alternating cycle of night and day. It puts us to sleep at night by secreting melatonin and wakes us up in the morning by stopping its flow. A deficiency in this hormone can prevent us from sleeping. This can be taken care of with melatonin supplements.

We think of hibernation in terms of animals spending the cold winter months in a deep sleep, but in fact we hibernate every night in the sense that while asleep, our organ functions slow and fall into disrepair.

Then when the sun rises in the morning, the pineal turns off the flow of melatonin, and our organ functions, immediately restored, speed up again.

SUGGESTIONS FOR INSOMNIA*

- ➤ **Lithium** (20 mg/day). Lithium works well for insomnia. Take it when all other remedies have failed.
- ➤ **Ginkgo biloba.** It not only helps induce sleep but also improves the quality of sleep. It's especially effective in cases of depression.
- ➤ **Intense light.** Designed to prevent SAD (seasonal affective disorder), intense light also promotes sleep (see Resources). Some people have to use the light device in the morning to avoid altering their biological clocks, which keeps them up at night. In some it induces sleep no matter when they use it.
- ➤ **Diet.** Avoid any foods that cause indigestion or stimulate the nervous system.
- ➤ **Thyroid supplements.** Take supplements to correct low thyroid function, which is one cause of sleep disorders (see Chapter 5).
- ➤ **Calcium (microcrystalline hydropoxidite), magnesium, and vitamin B$_6$.** Modest amounts of these nutrients induce sleep by calming the nerves.
- ➤ **Melatonin.** Take less than 1 mg right before going to bed.
- ➤ **Inositol** (100 mg/day).
- ➤ **Complete darkness.** Use an eye mask or completely opaque window dressing to normalize melatonin function.
- ➤ **Avoid antidepressants** or any other drug medication that prevents dreaming.

---

*Take as many as possible of these nutrients in the form of whole food complexes. For dosage, follow the directions on the label.

CHAPTER 14

ALCOHOLISM

Robert Dudley, a biologist at the University of Texas, writes that our liking for alcohol was passed on to us from our closest relatives on the evolutionary scale—chimpanzees, gorillas, and orangutans who traveled miles through dense forest thickets in search of fermented fruit. Dudley asserts that the purpose was to obtain "precious calories."[1] But why go to such lengths for fuel when fresh fruit containing plenty of sugar for the production of body energy was close at hand? I'm convinced these primates sought fermented fruit for the same reason that the Chinese ferment soybeans and the Eskimos and Hebrides Islanders devised ways of putrefying meat and fish—because eating foods partially broken down by bacteria increases energy, strengthens muscles, and improves digestion. A liking, then, among our primate relatives for the taste and euphoric effect of fermented fruit developed originally from the health benefits derived from it.

Addiction to alcoholic beverages among Europeans, who for most of their existence had been nomadic hunters and food gatherers, became a problem after they settled down to cultivate grains. Their digestive systems, used to handling meat protein, didn't have the enzymes needed to break down the protein in grains, particularly the gluten protein in wheat, rye, and barley. Those people who developed an allergy to certain grains, by extension, became allergic to the alcoholic drinks made from these grains. This led to an unnatural craving for alcohol.

Thus individuals today who crave alcohol prefer the alcoholic beverage that is made out of the grain or other food substance to which they are allergic—corn, wheat, barley, rye, potatoes, or grapes. Eating allergy-causing grains makes some individuals crave the alcoholic form of the grain because the acidic waste from the undigested grains in bread and cereals make them nervous and jumpy. Alcohol does away with these feelings by relaxing the nerves. Alcoholics are mistaken in thinking they're driven to drink only because they like the way it tastes and the feeling of relaxation and euphoria it gives them. All of this is true, but the root cause of their need to relax and enjoy the taste of alcohol is due to the "jitters" they get from the acidic waste by-products of the grains or other foods that they don't digest well or are allergic to. Dr. Theron G. Randolph, author of the four-day rotation diet, found that among forty drinkers, each one was allergic to the food product—corn, wheat, rye, grapes, or potatoes—from which the alcoholic beverage they preferred was made.

While meat eaters are more likely to become alcoholics if they eat a lot of foods made from grains, grain eaters are more vulnerable to alcoholism if they give up their ancestral dietary grain staple for red meat and cow's milk. This is because each cultural group has protein-digesting enzymes that have been shaped by the kinds of protein that served as their ancestors' dietary staple. I came across an example of this in a special education course I taught a few years ago. During a class discussion, Isabel, a teacher of handicapped children, talked about parental alcoholism as the cause of learning disabilities in children. She said that most of the parents of her students whom she had met had alcohol on their breath. This reminded her of her own battle with alcoholism, and she stayed after class to tell me her story.

Isabel came from Colombia, South America, and described herself as an indigenous person, a descendent of the ancient Inca Indians. She told me that among Indian families today in Colombia all the family members, even the small children, drink alcoholic beverages, with the result that most Indians are already alcoholics in childhood. Isabel, her second husband, and her two sons were all alcoholics, but, determined to give up drinking, they moved to the United States to get away from the alcoholic environment in which they were living. This didn't work, so they returned to Colombia and put themselves under the care of a healer, referred to by Isabel as a bio-energetic doctor. This doctor prescribed a number of herbs and outlined a diet designed to heal their body tissues, which the toxic by-products of alcohol had inflamed.

Foods that were forbidden because of their inflammatory tendency—due to the fact that they were not part of their natural diet—were cow's milk, meat, fruit, and tomatoes. The first week Isabel and her family were allowed only two foods: potato and pumpkin soup; the second week vegetables and brown rice were added; and the third week goat's milk to reduce inflammation caused by meat and cow's milk. Isabel, her husband, and her sons were also given vaccines against parasites, and the doctor swung a pendulum aligned with the liver to increase its flow of energy. Isabel's sons are still fighting alcoholism, but the diet made it possible for Isabel and her husband, an alcoholic schizophrenic, to give up drinking by eliminating their nervousness. Isabel stressed that it was the stabilization of her nervous system that took away her craving for drink—and cigarettes. Hearing this story, I was reminded that when I eat a food to which I'm allergic, I become nervous and restless until I go on an eating binge, which has the same relaxing effect on my nerves as a drinking spree has on the nerves of an alcoholic. Isabel's dietary treatment for her alcoholism was successful because it duplicated the grain (rice and quinoa), root vegetable, and goat's milk diet of her ancestors.

Acidic Waste Triggers Craving for Alcohol

How do acidic wastes from the by-product of alcohol and undigested food debris set up a craving for alcohol? With the continued consumption of allergy-causing foods, acid particles triggered by histamines pile up and acidify the blood. The increased acidification of the alkaline blood pH elicits a reaction from the adrenals. They speed up production of the stress-promoting hormones because hyperacidity is taken by the adrenals as a sign that the body's survival is threatened. (That's because anger and fear also raise blood acid levels.) But because in reality there is no danger, the individual's urge to be involved in some physical action has no outlet. This builds tension, which sets up a craving for anything—food, alcoholic beverages, caffeinated drinks, or cigarettes—that will relieve the pressure. Which addiction grabs hold of such individuals depends on where their physical vulnerability lies. While an alarm reaction, triggered by hyperacidity, initiates the descent into alcoholism, the craving for alcohol is strengthened whenever the alcoholic takes a drink and the liver can't neutralize the acid aldehyde by-product of the alcohol. This continual onslaught on the liver causes hangovers to become more severe—headaches, dizziness, irritability, trembling, and a lack of coordination. The deeper the hangover, the more intense the craving for alcohol, which explains why alcoholism becomes worse with time.

Alcohol and the Brain

After the liver, the brain is the next most vulnerable organ to the damaging effects of chronic alcohol consumption because its energy needs are greater than those of any other organ in the body. In advanced stages of alcoholism, the brain doesn't get the glucose and oxygen needed for the production of energy. The alcoholic liver is not able to supply the brain with these raw materials, and blockages in the small blood vessels prevent them from delivering energy-generating oxygen and glucose to the brain. These blockages occur because when the liver is no longer able to process acidic wastes, they accumulate in the blood and cause the red blood cells to stick together. Acidic waste in the blood also attracts bacteria that feed on it. The result is clumps of agglutinous material that clog the blood vessels throughout the body so that there is very little space in the blood for glucose, oxygen, and other nutrients. Without these raw materials needed to produce cellular energy and for the repair and regeneration of the cells, brain function breaks down and the neurons drown in their own metabolic waste.

There may be another factor in the brain of the alcoholic that prevents it from generating energy. The brains of hamsters, put on a diet of alcohol for experimental purposes, couldn't use glucose as a fuel, according to the scientist Mary Kay Roach, a colleague of chemist Roger Williams, who conducted the experiment.[2] This indicates that it isn't always a lack of glucose that prevents the alcoholic brain from meeting its energy needs but the inability of the brain to use it. However, there is a compound besides glucose that the brain can use for fuel, and that is L-glutamine. After it crosses the blood-brain barrier, L-glutamine is converted to glutamic acid. I suspect that the brain can use glutamic acid to manufacture energy because it reduces excess ammonia, a toxic compound (from the breakdown of amino acids) that probably destroys glucose before it has a chance to enter the brain cells and be oxidized. In *Nutrition Against Disease*, Roger Williams writes about several alcoholic individuals in which L-glutamine eliminated the craving for alcohol.[3]

The healing effects of both niacin and L-glutamine, obtained by the neutralization and elimination of acid waste and alien chemicals, serve as a reminder that toxicity—which is almost overwhelmingly acidic in nature—is the fundamental cause of alcoholism. But the addiction for alcohol manifests itself only if there is an adrenal weakness that causes wild swings in blood sugar and/or an enzyme deficiency that prevents the liver from breaking down the toxic by-products of alcohol. In many cases, however, these weaknesses cause alcohol addiction only when the diet is not compatible with the metabolism. An inappropriate or junk-food diet triggers the actions of adrenal hormones that disrupt the concentration and normal distribution of sugar—one of the most important factors in metabolic function. The first step, then, in a program designed to overcome alcoholism is for the individual to take the niacin self-test to find out whether to go on the meat eater's or grain eater's diet.

Cirrhosis of the Liver

Not only does putting the body on emergency alert (adrenal overstimulation) create anxiety and tension that drives some people to alcoholism, but it also starts a cycle of reactions that ultimately destroy the liver. The liver, responding to the alert from the adrenals to raise blood sugar levels, takes an excessive amount of glucose out of storage and releases it into the bloodstream. Because there is really no need for this sudden rise in blood sugar, an increase in insulin produced by the beta cells in the pancreas drastically lowers blood sugar levels, causing hypoglycemia (low blood sugar). Low blood sugar means sluggish energy production, which interferes with liver function. It can also cause fatigue and depression, symptoms that, like anxiety, increase the craving for alcohol. As long as the individual continues drinking and acid levels in the blood remain high, the adrenals will direct the liver to raise blood sugar excessively and insulin will respond by reducing it precipitously.

Eventually the liver can't comply with the adrenal hormones' request for more glucose because it no longer has any. (The liver stores glucose in the form of glycogen.) One reason for this is that the drinker, preferring alcohol to food, doesn't supply the liver with the carbohydrates, protein, and fat it needs to make glucose. Another is the presence of fat, which should pass out of the liver into general circulation but can't because of alcohol's destruction of the B vitamin choline. (The absence of choline prevents fat from being converted by the liver into phospholipids, which can pass through phospholipid molecules in the cellular membrane of the cells in the liver into the bloodstream.) So fat molecules, remaining in the liver and needing a place to park themselves, fill up the spaces in the liver that are designed to store glucose. Fatty deposits also replace liver cells that have been destroyed by the alcoholic by-product, acid aldehyde. As if that weren't enough, metabolic wastes and acid aldehyde inflame the liver by destroying oxygen. Inflamed tissue develops scars, just like a wound or incision does. But scar tissue on the surface of the skin is harmless, whereas scar tissue in the liver destroys its ability to function by impeding circulation. An almost nonexistent blood supply turns the liver tissue into hard fibers, a sign that the liver has developed cirrhosis, a disease that, without early nutritional intervention, is fatal.

Can the recovered alcoholic heal the brain damage caused by the brain's inability to generate energy? Studies conducted by researchers at the Massachusetts General Hospital and Boston University using MRI images reveal that long-term abstinence from alcohol does bring some cognitive recovery.[4] The most primitive part of the brain, however, never recovers. This is the limbic system, made up of the amygdala, where fear and aggression originate, and the hippocampus, where long-term memories are stored. The ability of the amygdala, even in the long-term abstinent alcoholic, to supply the necessary neurons that enable humans to recognize what facial expressions mean, is permanently lost. Yet giving up alcohol does result in the partial recovery of the most recently evolved part of the brain—the cerebral cortex.

SUGGESTIONS FOR ALCOHOLISM AND CIRRHOSIS*

➤ **Thyroid supplements.** Normalizing energy levels improves the liver's ability to detoxify and rebuild its tissues (see Chapter 5).

➤ **Vitamin E** (800 to 1,000 units/day). Take vitamin E to assist the thyroid supplements in improving thyroid function.

➤ **Take the niacin test and make appropriate changes in the diet.**

➤ **Far infrared heating pad or magnetic mattress pad and pillow.** Use these products to reduce acidic waste in the body; also try placing magnetic pads directly on the liver.

When symptoms have lessened, the following nutritional supplements can be gradually added:

➤ **Magnesium** (400 to 800 mg/day). This helps neutralize acids.

➤ **Choline** (250 mg four times daily). Fat can't pass out of the liver into the blood without choline. Alcohol destroys choline, which is why alcoholics have fatty livers.

➤ **B complex capsule.** Take a B complex three times daily.

➤ **Vitamin C** (1,000 mg/day).

➤ **L-glutamine** (one to four grains a day). L-glutamine picks up excess ammonia and converts it into glutamic acid. It is also used by the brain for energy.

➤ **Niacin** (3 to 10 g/day). Most alcoholics respond best to 6 g of niacin/day.

➤ **Acupuncture** (as often as needed). A Korean woman with cirrhosis of the liver, given only six months to live, was treated by an acupuncturist. Ten years after her first treatment she was still in good health.

*Take as many as possible of these nutrients in the form of whole-food complexes. For dosage, follow the directions on the label.

CHAPTER 15

PROSTATE PROBLEMS AND HORMONAL DYSFUNCTION

The health of the prostate begins to degenerate when the acid-alkaline ratio of its two principal hormones, testosterone and dihydrotestosterone, becomes imbalanced. These two hormones work together but also oppose each other. Dihydrotestosterone (DHT) promotes acidity while testosterone encourages alkalinity. It's the stress-promoting, acidic hormone, DHT, however, that rises excessively, causing the level of the life-promoting, alkaline testosterone to drop. When that happens, the acid-alkaline pH of the blood and lymph systems becomes too acidic.

What induces this imbalance in the middle-aged and older man? Surprisingly, it is less the acidic waste from poor digestion than the highly acidic pollutants from manufacturing plants that have been spewed into the air and water and have gotten into the food supply.

When men entering their forties begin putting on weight in the abdominal region, they notice their muscles have weakened, their shoulders have narrowed, they don't feel as energetic as they once did, and they sometimes feel "low." This is because the testosterone-dihydrotestosterone ratio is reversing. Testosterone levels have dropped because it is being converted to dihydrotestosterone. Elevated DHT is accompanied by increasing estrogen levels; together they increase acidity in the prostate and by doing so decrease its alkalinity. (Men and women have the same hormones, only in different ratios.)

During puberty estrogen and dihydrotestosterone also become elevated, but for a good reason. They stimulate the growth of cells that bring the penis, testicles, prostate, and secondary sexual characteristics to maturity. Once puberty is over and the usefulness of these hormones declines, testosterone is no longer converted to DHT, and estrogen levels fall. Then as men enter middle or older age, their hormone levels come to resemble the levels of their adolescent years. Testosterone again diminishes because an enzyme in the prostate, 5 alpha reductase, converts it to DHT, and estrogen levels inch up.[1]

High estrogen and DHT levels and a decline in testosterone—the culprits in prostate dysfunction—cause the excessive growth of prostate tissue, diminish the sex drive, and are responsible for fewer and less viable sperm being produced.[2]

Testosterone's influence extends far beyond the prostate. When testosterone levels drop, plaque begins to form in the arteries. Moreover, the drop in testosterone places the body on emergency alert. Excessively high DHT, along with estrogen, causes the adrenal hormones to become permanently elevated. This in turn causes the muscles, nerves, heart, and lungs to become chronically overactive, while depressed levels of alkaline-forming testosterone levels slow up the digestive process as well as the cyclical death and regenerating of cells. This gives rise to excessive acid waste by-products. The elevation of the stress-promoting estrogen is particularly lethal because it destroys oxygen. This causes the blood to clot, thyroid function to slow up, the alteration of fats and oils, and an increase in histamine levels. High dihydrotestosterone levels and low testosterone explain why, when a man's prostate becomes enlarged, he is also more likely to develop arthritis, become subject to low-grade infections, and lose vitality and sharpness of intellect.

TONY FINDS A CURE FOR HIS PROSTATE PROBLEM

In his late forties Tony began having difficulty urinating, and for the first time in his life he started getting up at night to go to the bathroom: first once a night, then twice, until finally he was getting up every hour. The doctor confirmed that he had an enlarged prostate. Because his prostate specific antigen (PSA) was zero, bacterial inflammation and cancer were ruled out. This left excess prostate tissue, referred to as benign prostate hypertrophy (BPH).

Tony took two capsules a day containing an herbal combination of red clover, pygeum, saw palmetto, stinging nettles, and goldenseal on my recommendation. I also recommended he take a zinc supplement, since more zinc is utilized by the prostate than any other organ and men with prostate enlargements usually have a zinc deficiency (there is eight times more zinc in the prostate than in any other organ), as well as vitamin B_6, which converts zinc into a form that can be absorbed by the prostate cells. Although nutritional supplements are less likely to shrink a prostate that has become enlarged because of BPH than from inflammation, Tony's prostate shrank after he had been taking supplements for two and a half months. He now gets up only twice a night. I recommended that Tony take raw, organic sunflower and pumpkin seeds and green tea instead of the herbal formula (see suggestions at the end of the chapter). His one remaining problem was to find a way to get back to sleep after he got up at night. The solution turned out to be melatonin, a hormone secreted by the pineal gland in the brain. Melatonin not only helped Tony get a better night's sleep, but it most likely also helped maintain the health of his prostate by making it easier for the prostate to absorb zinc.

Why Prostate Problems Have Become Epidemic

According to a paper published in *Grana Palynologica* in 1960 by Erik Ask-Upmark, M.D., of the University of Upsala in Sweden, an enlarged prostate was at that time considered a new pathological condition.[3] Curiously, the processing of flour, widespread by 1900, which removed nutrients vital to the prostate such as zinc, magnesium, and vitamin E, didn't cause an epidemic of prostatitis or benign prostate hypertrophy as it did coronary heart disease. That is because prostate enlargement has a different cause.

When enlarged prostate glands were first noted in 1960, insecticides such as DDT and chemical food additives had been in widespread use only for about ten years (the chemical industry didn't go into high gear until a few years after World War II had ended). By 1976, when 60 percent of the men over sixty in North America were found to have some prostate enlargement, insecticides and chemical food additives had been in use for about twenty-five years, enough time for these chemicals to have caused an epidemic of prostate problems in older men.

Medical researchers suspect that an increase in the enzyme 5 alpha reductase—the enzyme that triggers the excess growth of prostate tissue—is caused by pesticides and industrial solvents. The problem with these manufactured chemicals is that they can't be broken down in the digestive tract, deactivated by the liver, and excreted by the kidneys or lungs, so they're either stored in the liver or go back into the circulatory system. Along with acidic waste from undigested food, they are deposited by the circulating blood inside the tiniest capillaries, some of which carry oxygen and nutrients to the prostate. Furthermore, some of this toxic waste seeps out of these capillaries into the extracellular fluid surrounding the prostate and inflames it. The rest of it clogs the capillaries, which prevents the prostate from getting sufficient nutrients and oxygen. This partial cutoff of nutrients and oxygen is especially harmful to the prostate gland because of its poor blood supply. (This could explain why three amino acid supplements—alanine, glycine, and glutamic acid—are effective in reducing prostate enlargement, as Doctors H. M. Feinblatt and J. C. Gant found in their crossover study of patients with enlarged prostates.[4]) The connection between manufactured chemicals and the deterioration of the prostate gland in the majority of men over sixty in the past forty years points out the importance of avoiding food with chemical additives and of drinking distilled water.

The fact that it is elevated levels of estrogen and DHT that trigger the production of excess tissue in the prostate gland is what makes saw palmetto, pygeum, and pollen seeds effective in treating BPH. These herbs contain healthy hormones such as testosterone that reduce the levels of these two rogue hormones. They do so either by preventing the conversion of testosterone to DHT or by preventing DHT and estrogen from binding to the receptors (openings) of the prostate cells. Zinc, if taken with vitamin B_6, also prevents the enzyme 5 alpha reductase from converting testosterone to DHT. The resulting shrinkage of the prostate helps normalize urine flow and heal possible kidney damage caused by the pressure of the prostate gland on the kidneys.

However, the most effective treatment for prostate enlargement is taking the three amino acids mentioned earlier: alanine, glycine, and glutamic acid. These amino acids are present in prostate fluid. Although considered nonessential because the body makes them, it is safe to assume, given their great success in reducing enlarged prostates, that men with prostate problems are deficient in them. According to a recent, exhaustive study of subjects with prostate enlargement who took these three amino acids for two months, 92 percent had a reduction in the size of their prostate gland and 95 percent urinated less frequently at night.[5]

Side Effects of Nutritional Supplements and How to Avoid Them

While there are many supplements that reduce prostate swelling, they shouldn't be taken indiscriminately on the assumption that they have no side effects. It is vital that supplements taken to reduce enlargement of the prostate don't cause the enzyme 5 alpha reductase to fluctuate. The problem is that nutritional supplements that are good at reducing prostate enlargement also tend to either raise or lower the level of this enzyme. This can have dire health consequences.

Studies show that 5 alpha reductase levels can be lowered by taking saw palmetto, zinc, and especially the essential fatty acid alpha linolenic acid (ALA). All three of these supplements increase the risk of prostate cancer. A study published in the *Journal of the National Cancer Institute* found that men in the highest quartile of ALA intake had four times the risk of prostate cancer compared to those in the lowest quartile.[6]

Some nutritional supplements can have the opposite effect and raise the level of 5 alpha reductase. Raising levels of 5 alpha reductase excessively, like lowering them, can cause the prostate cells to mutate and become malignant.

There are two health products that can normalize 5 alpha reductase enzyme levels, thus doing away with the risk of prostate cancer. They are vitamin C and green tea. A colleague of mine had his prostate removed followed by a series of chemotherapy treatments. His doctors, pessimistic about his complete recovery because the cancer had spread to his lymph nodes, told him if he remained cancer-free for five years he could consider himself cured. He began drinking one cup of organic green tea every night before going to bed and has kept up the habit. It has been nine years since his prostate removal and chemotherapy treatments, and he is still cancer-free.

Increasing the Sex Drive in Men

In men and women the same hormones fuel the sex drive—progesterone, testosterone, estrogen, and DHEA; but they are proportioned differently. They also play different roles. For example, while progesterone is the chief hormone involved in the sex drive in women, testosterone is the hormone principally responsible for arousing men's sex drives. Men have on average forty to sixty times more testosterone than adult females. Testosterone in men, then, is the equivalent hormone to progesterone in women.

While the dominance of estrogen over progesterone in women lowers the sex drive, the conversion of testosterone to dihydrotestosterone (DHT) lessens the sex drive in men. Since testosterone drops 1 to 2 percent each year beginning at the age of thirty, men start out with a disadvantage. The lowering of the libido due to the conversion of testosterone to DHT by the enzyme 5 alpha reductase, however, can be slowed. Diet should be the first consideration.

Take the niacin test to establish your metabolic type—meat eater, grain eater, or balanced metabolism—and then follow through with the right diet. This will lower the acid waste in the blood that accelerates the conversion of testosterone to DHT and increases estrogen levels. Getting rid of abdominal fat is essential because the fat cells in the abdomen absorb testosterone. When this happens the body is robbed of the hormone that stimulates the sex drive and helps keep the body young. Omega-3, omega-6, and omega-9 fatty acids are necessary for testosterone production. Eating a variety of organic, unroasted nuts, including walnuts, is the best way to satisfy these fatty acid requirements.

Increasing the Libido

Injections of pure testosterone boost the libido, but a more effective way of taking testosterone is transdermally, such as patches or pellets implanted under the skin. Taking testosterone "in a steady day-in-day-out pattern doesn't make sense," according to Dr. Eugene Shippen, M.D., author of *The Testosterone Syndrome*. He writes that testosterone should be taken in some rhythmic pattern that reflects the peaks and valleys in which it is secreted in the body. But while he writes that in young men testosterone peaks every ninety minutes, what the alternating highs and lows of testosterone are in middle-aged and older men has apparently not yet been discovered.

Another remedy for low sex drive in men is DHEA, a hormone produced by the adrenals. (Soviet scientists found a significant relationship between a low serum level of DHEA and erectile dysfunction.) Use topical DHEA. It's useless to take DHEA by mouth. When it enters the body through the digestive system and is carried by the blood to the liver to be detoxified, the liver sends the hormones to the intestines where they are eliminated.

SUGGESTIONS FOR PROSTATE ENLARGEMENT*

➤ **Three amino acids: glycine** (50 mg), **alanine** (50 mg), and **glutamic acid** (50 to 100 mg). Take two capsules twice daily for ten to fourteen days, and then reduce to one capsule once or twice daily. This supplement should be accompanied by vitamin C and green tea to keep the 5 alpha reductase enzymes stable so as to reduce the risk of prostate cancer.

➤ **Thyroid supplements.** Take these to speed up the disposal of acidic wastes (see Chapter 5).

➤ **Pregnenolone** (1 to 5 mg/day). Go off every so often for one week.

➤ **Raw carrots.** Eat one or more raw carrots a day to reduce inflammation.

➤ **Vitamin B$_6$** (60 mg/day). B$_6$ must be taken with zinc to facilitate its absorption.

➤ **Unroasted (raw) organic sunflower seeds.** Store in a glass jar and keep in the refrigerator.

➤ **Pollen seed extract** (300 to 500 mg/day).

continued

➤ **Keep intake of foods with high levels of alpha linolenic acid (ALA) to a minimum.** This includes flaxseed, soybeans, canola oil, commercial salad dressings, and margarine.

➤ **Red clover extract** (50 mg/day).

➤ **Stinging nettles** (600 mg/day).

➤ **Pygeum** (200 mg/day).

➤ **Vitamin E** (800 to 1,600 units/day). Vitamin E is a prostate cancer preventive, according to a controlled study done in Finland that was coauthored by Dr. Demetrius Albanes of the National Cancer Institute.[7]

➤ **Caprylic acid** (400 to 1,000 mg/day). Take in buffered form, which is effective for prostate infections caused by yeast cells.

The following supplements are effective in reducing enlarged prostates but have been shown in studies to increase the risk of prostate cancer:

➤ **Zinc arginate** (45 to 60 mg/day).

➤ **Saw palmetto** (320 mg/day).

➤ **Alpha linolenic acid (ALA).**

---

*Take as many of these nutrients as possible in the form of whole-food complexes. Follow the directions on the label.

CHAPTER 16

FEMALE REPRODUCTIVE DISORDERS

There is an ongoing struggle in the body between such stress-promoting hormones as cortisol, adrenaline, epinephrine, and estrogen and life-enhancing hormones like progesterone, pregnenolone, and DHEA. When the stress hormones are chronically elevated—they increase with age, during times of mental stress, and as the result of a bad diet—they endanger life. They do so by lowering the levels of the life-promoting hormones.

Nowhere is this struggle for power between the life-promoting and death-promoting hormones more evident than in the female reproductive system. The antagonists are estrogen and progesterone, the system's two principal regulating hormones. When they are balanced they help maintain the equilibrium of the blood's pH. Estrogen increases blood acid levels and stimulates the production of lactic acid, while progesterone, by putting a break on estrogen's overproduction of acid, increases the blood's alkalinity.

Both hormones are generated by the cuplike follicle in which egg cells are encapsulated in the ovaries, but they function in opposite ways. Estrogen engineers the release of the egg into the fallopian tube (ovulation) and triggers the growth of nutrient-rich tissues in the uterus for the support of the anticipated entry of the fertilized egg into the uterus. Progesterone, referred to as the pregnancy hormone, maintains the nutritional needs of the fertilized egg (embryo) after it is attached to the uterine wall.

When estrogen and progesterone levels are normal, they act as a brake on each other to ensure balanced function. If progesterone, in an effort to ensure adequate nourishment of the fetus, raises blood sugar too high, estrogen triggers the production of additional insulin to take the excess glucose out of circulation. (The excess glucose is converted to fatty acid and stored in the adipose tissues.) Or if progesterone causes the metabolism of too much fatty acid, estrogen reduces it—thus lessening the risk of heart disease. On the other hand, when estrogen spurs an overgrowth of tissue and blood in the uterus, progesterone slows estrogen down.

Estrogen and progesterone are considered balanced in menstruating women if they adhere to the following rhythmic cycling: On the first three days of the menstrual month, both estrogen and progesterone levels are low. Then estrogen starts climbing until it reaches its highest point on day 12, in the middle of the menstrual month. This peak causes the discharge of an egg from the ovary (ovulation) and also triggers the flow of progesterone. Estrogen drops slightly while progesterone gradually rises until its peak is reached on day 21. Then it starts to fall. The drop in progesterone signals the body to start menstruating. Thus these two hormones work in tandem, seesawing back and forth. When one reaches its peak, it spurs the flow of the other, which is at its lowest ebb. In short, while estrogen and progesterone occasionally flow at the same rate, normally they fluctuate in opposite directions.

Overall health and the prevention of breast, uterine, endometrial, and ovarian cancer in menstruating women depends on maintaining the monthly rhythmic cycle of estrogen and progesterone. Yet it is out of balance in most women. The blame falls on many shoulders, including pesticides and other synthetic chemicals that have the same molecular structure as estrogen so that once inside the body they mimic estrogen's functions, in effect, increasing the body's overload of estrogen.

Other factors that increase estrogen levels, thus upsetting the monthly estrogen-progesterone cycle, are toxic wastes that thicken the blood so that there is not enough space for vital nutrients to be transported to the reproductive system; poor diet; late-life pregnancies; the rejection of breast feeding in favor of formula; and mental stress, which, by raising blood levels of cortisol, causes estrogen levels to rise.

With estrogen sky high, progesterone, even in some young women, is nonexistent. Without progesterone, ovulation does not occur, and pregnancy is no longer possible. Worse still, with progesterone levels at zero, its protective effect against cancer is lost.

When women show premenstrual or perimenopausal symptoms such as irritability, fatigue, headaches, inertia, and so on, indicating their estrogen-progesterone cycle is imbalanced, doctors are apt to pre- scribe hormone replacement therapy (HRT), a combination of estrogen synthesized from the urine of the mare horse, and progestin, a syn- thetic form of progesterone. Progestin's molecular structure is different from that of the naturally occurring progesterone in the body. Legions of studies show the bad effects of this synthetic hormone medication. The progestin in HRT as well as in birth control pills increases the risk of breast and ovarian cancer as well as heart disease. One study done in Europe, with more than eighty thousand postmenopausal women, found that those who took progestin along with estrogen for an average of eight years had a 70 percent higher risk of breast cancer than those who took the bio-identical form of progesterone or didn't use hormones at all.[1]

What is the solution, besides the obvious—improving the diet and exercising? It is the replacement of synthetic progestin with natural progesterone, and estrogen derived from horses' urine with estrogen derived from herbs and other plant foods. T. S. Wiley, an anthropolo- gist specializing in endocrinology in molecular medicine and genetics, is conducting a study using bio-identical hormones according to the normal estrogen-progesterone monthly cycling pattern.[2] The theory behind rhythmic cycling is that, no matter how old a woman is, if her intake of natural estrogen/progesterone mimics the monthly rhythmic cycle of these hormones in menstruating women, the brain will think she is menstruating and therefore still fertile. According to Wiley, this causes the brain to conclude that her life is worth saving. It sends this message to the rest of the body, with the result that the organ systems begin to function the way they did when the body was young.

The problem with Wiley's rhythmic cycling is that it adds to the overload of estrogen in the body. It might be conducive to a long and healthy life if it weren't for the fact that, living in an estrogen-polluted world, everyone is supersaturated with this female hormone.

Estrogen's role in the attachment of the fertilized egg to the uterine wall helps explain why, during the rest of the individual's lifetime, estrogen, if excessive, is cancer threatening. The trouble starts at conception. The newly fertilized egg, the size of a speck of dust, must be attached instantly to the uterine wall or it will fall out of the uterus through the cervix. Once the embryo is attached, its nutritional needs must be met just as quickly. Trophoblastic cells in the embryo, triggered into action by estrogen, serve this purpose. Multiplying at a tremendously fast rate, they hook the embryo into the wall of the uterus, create half the placenta (the uterus creates the other half), and form the umbilical cord, which attaches the embryo to the placenta, the source of its food supply. Trophoblastic cells are able to grow like wild in the uterus because they can generate energy without oxygen. Estrogen makes this possible by lowering uterine oxygen levels. When the embryo has been in the uterus for seven or eight weeks, the work of the trophoblastic cells comes to an end and they migrate to the embryo's ovaries, if female, and testicles, if the embryo is male. There, they are converted by enzymes into germ cells (egg or sperm cells).

This is not necessarily the end of the trophoblastic cells, however. The germ cells can be converted back into trophoblastic cells any time estrogen levels become excessive. What is frightening about this is that trophoblastic cells multiply as fast as cancer cells. In fact, according to biochemist Dr. Ernst F. Krebs Jr., who studied seventeen thousand research experiments on the subject, trophoblastic cells are identical in all respects to cancer cells.[3] Three obvious similarities are the way in which the fingerlike projections of trophoblastic cells invade the uterine wall to implant the fetus, the speed with which they multiply, and the fact that trophoblastic cells, like cancer cells, generate energy without oxygen.

When estrogen is elevated, like all other chemicals in the body that are in excess, it no longer reacts according to the body's needs. It can create an oxygen-poor environment anywhere in the body at any time. If oxygen deprivation is severe enough, it causes cancer, because without oxygen, normal cells cannot generate energy. In order to survive, they convert into trophoblastic/cancer cells so they can generate energy anaerobically (without oxygen). If estrogen levels in the blood remain high with the result that estrogen destroys oxygen, the cancerlike trophoblastic cells keep on multiplying and a tumor forms.

Many studies confirm the role of estrogen in causing cancer. Dr. Ross Trattler, in *Better Health Through Natural Healing*, writes about a study linking synthetic estrogen therapy to a five- to twelvefold increase in uterine and breast cancer.[4] Two other studies provide additional evidence of the cancer-causing effects of synthetic hormones. One study found that estrogen therapy without progesterone causes a fourteenfold increase in endometrial cancer. The other study, published in the *Journal of the American Medical Association*, January 26, 2000, especially significant because it tracked 46,355 women, found that those who took HRT made up of synthetic hormones for five years were 40 percent more likely to develop breast cancer than women who were not on HRT.[5]

Doctors prescribe synthetic HRT not only to ease menopausal symptoms but also to prevent osteoporosis in menopausal and post-menopausal women. This is truly a double-edged sword. Any organ deprived of oxygen by the estrogen in HRT will absorb calcium, which hardens it. Thus while HRT may be successful in hardening the bones, it also hardens organs made of soft tissues. The consequences of the longtime use of HRT then is stronger bones and the hardening (degeneration) of the soft-tissue organs.

Breast Cancer Prevention

A significant factor in the cause of breast cancer is a deficiency in a type of vitamin D, called 25-hydroxy (vitamin D_3). Increasing your blood levels of 25-hydroxy D is imperative and when possible should be accomplished through exposure to sunlight rather than through supplements, since supplemental vitamin D is not absorbed well.[6]

Although *homo sapiens* (starting with Cro-Magnan man) have been around for at least fifty thousand years, it has been for only six to seven thousand years that most human population clusters have spent much time indoors. No wonder our metabolism works most efficiently if the vitamin D_3 in our bodies is produced by sunlight rather than from a capsule. That we haven't yet adapted to the artificial light in our indoor environment is revealed in the many studies that show that the less time women spend in the sun, the more likely they are to get breast cancer. (This also goes for multiple sclerosis in both men and women). Studies show that being exposed to sunlight is particularly important during adolescence and pregnancy, when breast tissue is growing. Women who had outdoor jobs between the ages of ten and forty have a 40 percent reduced risk of breast cancer.[7]

Many studies confirm the value of sunlight by showing that normal and above-normal blood levels of vitamin D are a protection against cancer. This reminds me of a cancer cure that received a lot of publicity more than thirty years ago. Because he had advanced cancer, William Ott, a photographer, went to Florida where the sun shines all year long. He sat in the sun every day from sunrise to sunset—until his cancer had completely disappeared.

It stands to reason that exposing yourself to the sun frequently could be a deterrent to the growth of cancer cells since the sun is the source of all our energy. If you can't spend time outdoors regularly, take two tablespoons of cod liver oil a day, one in the morning and the other in the evening after meals. Failing your ability to acquire a taste for cod liver oil, take 1,000 to 2,000 units of oil-based vitamin D_3 daily, preferably in the form of a whole-food vitamin supplement. Keep in mind that nothing can beat the health-giving power of sunshine.

The herb black cohosh also reduces the risk of breast cancer. According to a study carried out by Dr. Timothy R. Rebbeck at the University of Pennsylvania School of Medicine, it lowers the incidence of breast cancer by 53 percent. The study compared 949 healthy women with 1,524 women with breast cancer.[8]

Black cohosh works by reducing estrogen levels and has been shown to block cancer cell growth, according to Rebbeck. It could be that the lowered estrogen prevents cancer cells in the breast from growing. There is some anecdotal evidence that black cohosh also lowers blood insulin levels. Insulin, when excessively high, stimulates the recurrence of breast cancer.

Health Problems Associated with Estrogen Imbalance

The following female reproductive problems are nearly always related to excess estrogen and the concurrent drop in progesterone and oxygen. Estrogen-progesterone imbalance, however, does more than put a monkey wrench in the smooth functioning of the cyclical female reproductive cycle. It also imbalances the autonomic nervous system, which regulates all the organ systems—including the female reproductive organs. Thus a balance between estrogen and progesterone is vital for overall well-being as well as for normal functioning of the female reproductive system.

Infertility and Heavy Periods

When estrogen lowers energy levels by destroying oxygen, the pituitary can't produce the follicle-stimulating hormone and, as a result, follicles are not produced. When not encased in a follicle, egg cells cannot be released. And when ovulation doesn't occur, not only is pregnancy impossible but there is a buildup of the uterine lining that causes heavier and more frequent periods. Failure to ovulate is a sign that progesterone levels have dropped to zero.

Dr. Ben C. Campbell and Dr. Peter T. Ellison of Harvard University reported on a study of eighteen premenstrual women that revealed excess estrogen as the main cause of a drop in progesterone. Progesterone levels were checked in the middle of the menstrual cycle.[9] It was found that seven of the eighteen women in the study did not ovulate. While the numbers in this study are too small to draw any firm conclusions about progesterone deficiency, the prevalence of premenstrual symptoms in the female population is a sure sign of a progesterone shortage. The symptoms of PMS—water retention, fibrocystic breasts, depression, wrinkled skin, vaginal dryness, irregular and heavy periods— are the result of estrogen dominance over progesterone. The natural decrease of progesterone with age doesn't help matters. It drops to nearly zero at menopause, whereas estrogen simply decreases—anywhere from 40 percent to 60 percent. When the ovaries stop producing progesterone with the result that estrogen levels rise, there is a greater danger of getting heart disease and cancer.

Endometriosis

The lowering of oxygen levels by excess estrogen in the uterus increases acidity. The sharp acid crystals irritate and inflame the lining of the uterus. If oxygen deprivation is sustained, it results in endometriosis, inflammation of the uterine lining. When inflammation is chronic, the lining disintegrates and the fragments are carried by fluids to the ovaries, where they cause adhesions and cysts to form. Intercourse during menstruation can exacerbate endometriosis because it pushes mucus and blood up the uterus and fallopian tubes into the ovaries.

SUGGESTIONS FOR PMS AND ENDOMETRIOSIS*

➤ **Progesterone.** The most effective treatment for both PMS and endometriosis is progesterone. Take natural progesterone in the form of a topical cream. Apply once or twice a day in the areas where the blood vessels are close to the skin: the neck, the wrists, and inside the elbows. Take time off from this hormone the last two weeks of the menstrual cycle or, if you are postmenopausal, use it no more than three weeks out of every month.

➤ **Fatty acid blood profile.** This profile indicates possible deficiencies in alpha linolenic acid (ALA), although too much ALA has been implicated in prostate cancer; linoleic acid (LA); deoxyribonucleic acid (DHA); gamma linoleic acid (GLA); and arachidonic acid (AA). Primrose oil, which contains GLA fatty acid, has relieved PMS symptoms. Michael Schmidt in his book *Smart Fats* states that British studies show GLA relieves menstrual tension in 90 to 95 percent of cases. Meat eaters, however, should limit the quantity of polyunsaturated fatty acids in their diet. (See Resources.)

➤ **Avoid milk.** Milk is linked to a variety of reproductive disorders because the mucus it generates blocks the fallopian tubes.

➤ **Thyroid supplements.** A slightly above-normal thyroid function (as indicated by a temperature slightly higher than 98.6 degrees) helps relieve PMS and endometriosis by getting rid of acidic wastes in the body (see Chapter 5).

> ➤ **Avoid caffeine** in coffee, tea, chocolate, and cola soft drinks.
> ➤ **Black cohosh, valerian, and wild yam roots.** These contain hormones that normalize estrogen and progesterone levels.

*Take as many as possible of these nutrients in the form of whole-food complexes. For dosage, follow the directions on the label.

Miscarriages

High estrogen levels trigger miscarriages for a number of reasons. The most obvious is that excess estrogen causes excessive bleeding in the uterus during pregnancy. One of estrogen's functions during pregnancy is to reduce oxygen in the uterus so that fast-growing cells that generate energy anaerobically (without oxygen) can instantly attach the embryo to the uterine wall. But when estrogen levels are excessive it devours so much oxygen that there is not enough left over for the embryo. Professor Soderwell and his students at the University of Oregon found that miscarriage in older women was caused not by their older ova but rather by the unsuitability of the uterus.[10] Excessive estrogen's destruction of oxygen in the uterus could very well be why Soderwell's ova could not be implanted in the uterine wall.

Fibroid Uterine Tumors and Cystic Breasts

When estrogen levels are normal, after the menstrual period has ended, estrogen causes the uterine wall to rebuild its tissue in preparation for the possibility that the next egg released in the fallopian tube will be fertilized. Excess estrogen, however, overstimulates the growth of tissue in the uterus, sometimes creating such a thick uterine lining that it fails to disintegrate when the egg is not fertilized. Without impregnation, one layer of tissue is laid over another in the uterus. The hard, fibrous tissue thickens and forms a tumor. It seems probable, since elevated estrogen causes the growth of excess tissue in the uterus, that hormone replacement therapy containing estrogen extracted from horse urine has increased the number of women with uterine fibroid tumors. Of the six women I know who are on synthetic HRT, four have developed fibroid uterine tumors. Excessive estrogen also spurs the growth of breast tissue when it is not needed for lactating purposes, causing cysts to develop in the breasts.

Low Blood Sugar

Another of estrogen's functions during pregnancy is to lower excessive blood sugar. When levels of estrogen become elevated, it depresses blood sugar even when blood sugar levels are normal. If this happens during pregnancy, the fetus is deprived of the glucose necessary for normal development. Estrogen-induced low blood sugar may also be one reason why far more women than men suffer from depression and insomnia.

The most important factor in normalizing estrogen levels is to improve liver function, since it disposes of excess estrogen. This can be done, first, by working out a diet that produces the least amount of acidic waste. That way the liver, not having to expend so much energy neutralizing acid waste, can use its energy instead to dispose of estrogen. The ability of the liver to rid the body of estrogen, however, is also dependent on protein, so if your estrogen levels are excessive, those nutrients that metabolize protein should be taken: the amino acid methionine; vitamins B_1, B_2, E, C, and A; and natural thyroid extract. These nutrients, in addition, are the raw materials that convert cholesterol molecules into progesterone. An increase in progesterone lowers

---

EXCESS ESTROGEN CAN BECOME A LIABILITY IN WOMEN WHO ARE NOT PREGNANT

Estrogen lowers the expectant mother's immune system during pregnancy to prevent it from rejecting the fetus. When estrogen levels rise too high in women who are not pregnant, it has the same immune-lowering effect.

estrogen levels, and Vitamin E counteracts estrogen's destruction of oxygen by its oxygenating effects.

Another way to balance estrogen and progesterone levels is to stimulate the function of the pineal gland. The pineal, in the middle of the brain, delays puberty by lowering estrogen levels. It also wakes us up in the morning by absorbing sunlight and brings on sleep when darkness triggers its secretion of melatonin. By sleeping in as dark a room as possible at night and getting plenty of sunlight during the day, we can ensure that the pineal gland's ability to reduce estrogen increases and that it may become permanent. To obtain maximum benefit from the sunlight, try panning. Raise your head toward the sun, close your eyes, and move your head slowly to the left and then to the right, back and forth for at least five minutes at a time. When the sky is overcast, you can pan in front of a high-intensity light (see Resources). Even an ordinary lightbulb will bring results. To increase exposure to darkness during sleep, wear an eye mask, preferably padded, to keep out as much light as possible.

Health Consequences Associated with the Removal of Ovaries

The data from a study of 29,380 women, 16,345 of whom had a hysterectomy including removal of the ovaries, while the remaining 13,035 didn't have their ovaries removed when they had their uterus removed, was analyzed. It revealed that after twenty-four years those who had their ovaries removed were 12 percent more likely to have died, 17 percent more likely to develop lung cancer, and 17 percent more likely to get heart disease than those whose ovaries were left intact. Furthermore, their chances of getting Parkinson's disease doubled.[11] These are scary statistics as three hundred thousand women who have hysterectomies yearly also have their ovaries removed. The ostensible reason for their removal is to prevent ovarian cancer. Since, however, only 34 of the 13,035 women who kept their ovaries died of ovarian cancer, the removal of the ovaries, unless there is a family history of ovarian cancer, does not appear to be justified.

It may be possible to reduce fatalities from ovarian cancer if women are made aware of one of its early symptoms—digestive problems, such as nausea or acid reflux, unexplained weight gain, abdominal pain, or bloating. If you've had digestive problems for years, it is unlikely that they are a symptom of ovarian cancer. But if you've had no problem with indigestion, and then it hits you out of the blue, see your doctor immediately to have an MRI of your ovaries. Digestive disorders may occur at such an early stage of ovarian cancer that the removal of the ovaries can stop the cancer from spreading.

Fertility and Enhanced Sex Drive

Besides all the health problems caused by excessive estrogen—it suppresses immune reaction, destroys oxygen and blood sugar, causes heart attacks, increases the risk of cancer—it also depresses the sex drive.[12] At one time it was assumed that the libido was triggered by estrogen. It is now known that progesterone is the hormone that in women is most responsible for sexual feelings. (To a smaller extent, testosterone and DHEA are also involved in stimulating interest in sex.)

It is said that all feelings of sexuality originate in the brain. This makes sense in the case of women in view of the fact that progesterone levels in the brain are twenty times higher than in the blood.[13]

Progesterone not only enhances the sex drive but also boosts intelligence by increasing brain activity, regulates blood sugar, has a calming effect, prevents cancer (probably by building up the immune system), builds bone and thus protects against arthritis and osteoporosis, and neutralizes environmental toxins.

Because progesterone contributes to the overall wellness of the body as well as to its sexuality, whereas estrogen, because there is almost always too much of it, endangers health, it is important to get the blood levels of your hormones tested. (Mainstream medicine never tests progesterone levels!) Use the saliva test rather than the blood test to measure your progesterone levels because progesterone levels fluctuate. Progesterone is deficient in the vast majority of women. They should use a natural progesterone transdermal cream, preferably extracted from yams (see "Suggestions to Enhance the Sex Drive"). Another way to increase progesterone levels is to have eggs every day, liver once a week, and a lot of butter.

SUGGESTIONS TO ENHANCE THE SEX DRIVE

➤ **Progesterone cream** (for topical use). Apply to the wrists, the neck, or inside the elbows. Go off periodically. Menstruating women should apply the progesterone cream the last two weeks of the menstrual month, and postmenapausal women three weeks out of four.

➤ **Macca Pause** (made by Feminessence). This is an herb that, in some women, converts into progesterone.

➤ **Eggs daily, butter, and liver once a week.** These foods help increase progesterone production.

TIMOTHY AND MAUREEN: THEIR STRUGGLE TO HAVE A BABY

Timothy and Maureen badly wanted children, but the chances of Maureen becoming pregnant were slim. They were married when both were thirty-five. From the age of thirty on, there is a slight drop each year in fertility in both sexes. By age thirty-five, the chances of becoming pregnant plummet. Maureen's age was not the only factor making it difficult for her to become pregnant; a more serious liability was the fact that she ovulated only twice a year, so there were only two short periods in the year when she was fertile. These two difficulties were compounded by the fact that neither Maureen nor Timothy had much interest in sex.

Testosterone, although the principal male hormone, is also present in females and can stimulate the sex drive in women as well as in men. Testosterone levels can be boosted by taking a precursor hormone called pregnenolone, which converts into testosterone. Maureen and Tim took pregnenolone, extracted

continued

from yams. Pregnenolone can also be produced in the body by taking vitamins E and A, thyroid extract, and copper and sitting in front of a high-intensity light for a half hour each day, which is what Maureen and Timothy did. Both experienced an increase in their libido.

Four months after they went on this regimen, Maureen became pregnant. To avoid miscarriage and ensure that her blood nutrient levels were maintained, she took a natural form of progesterone. Nine months and two weeks after she became pregnant, Maureen gave birth to a healthy baby girl.

Nutritional Requirements for Conception, Pregnancy, and Breast Feeding

Of great importance in the effort to conceive, to sustain pregnancy, and to give birth to healthy and intelligent babies is the body's production of energy. Like eating for two and breathing for two, the pregnant woman must also produce enough energy for two—her own needs and the needs of the developing fetus. A vitally important factor in this matter is getting out every morning or late afternoon when the sun is at an angle. Even on overcast days, the sun shines through the clouds. Light increases the actions of the respiratory (energy-producing) enzymes. And the red spectrum of light that the sun emits is absorbed by the copper inside the cells' energy-producing factories, the mitochondria.

This shows that red light is directly involved in generating energy. The animal world knows more about how to make energy than we do. They go to great lengths to ensure their offspring are exposed to the maximum amount of light by migrating to regions where the days are longer during the mating season, gestation, and birth.

A diet geared to the maximum benefit of prospective offspring should begin three to six months before the attempt to conceive and should be compatible with the metabolism of the prospective mother. This will keep toxic acidic waste in the blood to a minimum so as not to raise estrogen levels, which can cause miscarriage. The prospective mother should eat foods that will satisfy the nutritional requirements of the fetus. The prime consideration should be extra sugar because higher-than-average blood sugar levels are necessary for the production of sufficient energy to sustain the growth of the fetus. Vitamins E and A as well as magnesium help maintain normal blood sugar, as does the appestat mechanism, by causing the expectant mother to crave sweets.

The craving for sweets should be satisfied by eating fruit. Not only is the fructose in fruit healthier than refined white sugar, but all fruits are rich in potassium. Potassium in the blood acts like insulin, facilitating the entry of sugar molecules into cells where they are used to produce energy. Potassium also removes sugar from the blood without causing blood sugar levels to drop precipitously the way elevated insulin does. When insulin levels are high (caused by the overconsumption of white sugar and refined carbohydrates) it lowers blood levels of calcium and phosphorus, which are needed to build the bones of the developing fetus. The old adage "a tooth lost for every child" acknowledges the draining of calcium reserves from the maternal blood supply. A study done in Norway confirms that in the later months of pregnancy, blood calcium levels become deficient.[14] A highly mineralized water helps make up for the loss of alkaline minerals during pregnancy and also helps maintain the alkaline pH of the blood.

Another important dietary measure during pregnancy is an increase in fats. The expectant mother's body relies increasingly on fat for its energy needs since the fetus uses up her supply of blood sugar and also because fatty acids in the maternal blood are used in the synthesis of the fetus's cellular membranes. What kinds of fats should the gestating woman eat?

The commonly held belief that most people are deficient in omega-3 fish oil is being shattered by the latest fatty acid research, conducted by Dr. Patricia Kane, a researcher at the Body-Bio Corporation (the Body-Bio Corporation tests fatty acid blood levels). It reveals there is a growing deficiency of omega-6 fats in many people due to the avoidance of meat fat, butter, and eggs in an effort to lower cholesterol. While omega-6 polyunsaturated oils such as corn, cottonseed, sesame, sunflower, and canola should not be consumed during pregnancy because they lower blood sugar, organic meat fat, raw egg yolk, and butter are good for building healthy fetuses. The supersaturated coconut oil is also good for the fetus because it normalizes energy production and is itself a good source of energy. Green, leafy vegetables are important as a source of omega-3 fatty acids.

Although saltwater fish is the best source of the docosahexaenoic acid (DHA), an omega-3 fatty acid, the Food and Drug Administration warns that women who are pregnant or planning to become pregnant should avoid shark, swordfish, king mackerel, tuna, and tilefish because they contain enough mercury to harm the developing fetus's brain. Salmon, mackerel, sardines, and anchovies are not on this list and are even better sources of DHA fatty acid.

High fat consumption during pregnancy, while vital to the fetus, has one drawback; it destroys vitamin B_6. This is one of many reasons it is necessary to consume plenty of quality protein, especially red meat with its whole range of B vitamins. Besides the use of protein as a building block of the body, its supply of B_6 replaces what is destroyed by high fat levels. Choline, another B vitamin, which is plentiful in meat, enhances the fetus's memory by altering the hippocampus, the memory center of the brain, according to researchers at the University of North Carolina at Chapel Hill.[15]

The B vitamins also play a key role in normalizing excessive hormone levels. Pantothenic acid destroys excess insulin, and when insulin levels fall, estrogen levels also drop. If high levels of insulin and estrogen in the maternal blood are absorbed into the fetal blood system, "they may alter mammary tissue in such a way that it responds to estrogen during puberty by becoming malignant," according to an article in the *New York Times* by Lawrence K. Altman.[16] The normalization of estrogen and insulin during pregnancy may prevent cancer after birth. A study conducted by Pamela J. Goodwin, M.D., found that women with breast cancer and high insulin levels were eight times more likely to die of breast cancer than those with breast cancer who had low insulin levels. One way of preventing breast cancer while at the same time building the intelligence and immune system of your baby is to breast-feed for two years or longer. According to a Yale University study of women in rural China, this reduces the chance of developing breast cancer by 50 percent.[17]

Nina Planck, author of the book *Real Food: What to Eat and Why*, wrote an excellent article in the *New York Times* about the dangers of a vegan diet for children as well as pregnant and nursing women.[18] Planck points out that vegetarian societies always included cheese, butter, and eggs in their diet—that in fact no vegetarian culture has ever existed that has excluded products derived from animals for the simple reason that there is not enough protein or fat in grains and other plants to supply all the necessary nutrients. No individual could survive into old age if his or her mother was on a vegan diet during pregnancy and while breast-feeding and then that individual was kept on a vegan diet through his or her teenage years.

Only animal protein and fats have all the essential amino acids and fatty acids. Furthermore, vitamin B_{12} is found only in animal foods. A baby and growing child needs plenty of protein and calcium. Soy, a food vegans use as a replacement for milk and animal protein, inhibits the absorption of protein and minerals.

Nutritional Supplements During Pregnancy

Besides the right diet, pregnant women should take a prenatal vitamin that is a whole-food complex. In all prenatal vitamins, the B vitamin content is too low with the exception of folic acid, so it's advisable to take extra B vitamins. Folic acid, the most important B vitamin, is not easy to absorb. To ensure your body's ability to utilize this vitamin, which prevents spina bifida and other birth defects, take 1 mg of methyl folate, the active form of folic acid. Don't take a prenatal vitamin that contains iron, since the liver has no way of excreting excess iron. Taking iron is also not a good idea because it destroys vitamin E. An additional supplement containing vitamin E is necessary since the amount of E in prenatal supplements is not sufficient. Also, a woman whose thyroid tests underactive should take thyroid supplements, preferably a natural thyroid supplement (see Chapter 5). If progesterone levels are too low—take a saliva test to determine your progesterone level—a natural progesterone cream should be used. Avoid caffeine during pregnancy. One to three cups of coffee a day increases the risk of miscarriages by 30 percent, according to a study conducted jointly by Sweden and the United States of 562 women who had miscarriages six to twelve weeks into pregnancy.[19]

SUGGESTIONS FOR PRECONCEPTION, PREGNANCY, LACTATION, AND GENERAL REPRODUCTIVE HEALTH*

➤ **Methyl folate** (1 mg/day). This is the active form of folic acid.

➤ **Progesterone.** Use natural progesterone topical cream, depending on the results of the saliva test. The offspring of mothers who take natural progesterone before pregnancy have a lower incidence of birth defects than the average. And those who take progesterone during pregnancy have babies who, in standardized tests, rank in the outstanding category.[20]

➤ **Vitamin E** (400 to 1,200 units/day).

➤ **Vitamin A** (10,000 to 25,000 units/day).

➤ **Vitamin D** (400 to 1,000 units/day). Thousands of units of vitamin D a day are reported to be safe. However, since one study shows long-term use of high-dosage vitamin D causes hardening of the arteries, take vitamin D in a whole-food complex.

➤ **Vitamin B$_6$** (250 to 500 mg/day).

➤ **Magnesium** (400 to 1,200 mg/day).

➤ **Zinc** (50 mg/day).

➤ **Vitamin C** (500 mg/day).

➤ **Calcium lactate** (400 to 800 mg/day).

*Take as many as possible of these nutrients in the form of whole-food complexes. For dosage, follow the directions on the label.

CONCLUSION

Scientists have led us to believe that good health and longevity are largely a matter of luck, that we are hostages to the genes handed down to us by our ancestors. The discovery that some people have genetic markers for particular diseases would appear to confirm this belief. But surprisingly, statistical research shows that many people with a gene predisposing them to, for example, breast cancer or insulin-dependent diabetes are not much more likely to come down with the disease than people who don't carry the genetic marker. The fact is that most disease-carrying genes need a trigger to become active. That trigger is acidic waste, largely the leftover remains of undigested foods.

If we describe health as the balance between two opposites—the way every healing system except modern medicine defines it—we would assume that a state of health exists in anyone whose acid and alkaline balances are normal. Yet it is possible to have normal pH of the blood, lymph, urine, and digestive juices and still be seriously ill.

That there is often no connection between an imbalance in the pH of the blood and the level of acid waste in the digestive tract or the state of health in a particular individual is not surprising, for toxic wastes and body chemicals are not dispersed evenly throughout the body. For example, tests can show a low level of heavy metal contaminants in the blood even when there is an excessive amount of heavy metal in the solid tissues of the body. There is even less of a connection between the pH of the blood and the ratio of acidic foods (foods with more acidic than alkaline particles) to alkaline foods (food with more alkaline than acid particles) in the diet. That too high a level of acidic minerals in foods is the cause of degenerative disease is disproven by the fact that tribal cultures whose dietary staple is grain—widely considered to be acidic because of its high level of phosphorous—are generally healthy and long-lived.

In fact, the real problem with domesticated grains is that, introduced into the diet at a fairly recent date in human history, not everyone's digestive system has had time to adapt to them.

When we eat a form of protein that our digestive system can't handle, it ends up as undigested acid waste. Acid waste creates an acid-alkaline imbalance by increasing blood levels of stress-related hormones such as cortisol and estrogen.

Balancing organ function and avoiding degenerative disease depends upon generating as little acidic waste as possible. The first priority is to avoid misconceptions as to what constitutes a healthy diet. Before the 1960s, when the cholesterol mania began, planning a diet around a "balanced" meal—protein, carbohydrates, and fat—was the gospel preached by the medical establishment. This credo not only fooled the public into assuming that a standardized diet was good for everyone, it also ignored the fact that refined flour and sugar and canned, over-cooked food, all part of this so-called balanced diet, had very little nutritional value.

The diet of the hunter-forager, a way of life now practically extinct, was the ideal. Eating animals and plants that grew wild in nature, much of it raw or, in the case of meat and fish, barely singed over a wood-burning fire, provided enough enzymes to convert the exact amount of digested food molecules needed for the repair and rebuilding of the body's cells, and no more. This guaranteed a slim and healthy body.

But emulating the diet of the hunter to the extent that it is possible in today's world is only part of the answer. The other part is finding foods that your body can handle. Testing yourself to find out what types of protein and vegetables you should eat and, when necessary, testing for food allergies is a good start, but awareness of how your body reacts to the foods you eat is even more important. The key to good health is to keep track of the foods you ate before you began to feel unwell and avoid them in the future. Only then can you be sure that your body is not producing too much acidic waste—the cause of all degenerative disease.

RESOURCES

Air cleaner. The Living Air Classic, ecoquest.com.

Alkaline water. Alka Life, 888-261-0870.

Castor oil therapy. Edgar Cayce products, 800-862-2923; The Heritage, Dept. C, P.O. Box 444, Virginia Beach, VA 23458-0444.

Cetyl myristate. For arthritis, high blood pressure, and fibromyalgia. Willner's Chemists, 800-633-1106.

Far infrared sleeping mat. Includes negative ions and pulsed magnetic fields. Transformation Technologies, 877-287-0912.

Fatty acid blood profile. Body-Bio Corporation, Dr. Patricia Kane, 856-8258-338.

Frequency Specific Microcurrent (FSM) device. For macular degeneration. frequencyspecific.com, 877-695-7500; altmedsales .com, 800-539-1320.

Gelatin (made from chicken or beef). For digestion problems, diabetes, and rebuilding cartilage. Bernard Jensen, 800-755-4027.

Glutathione (intravenous). For Parkinson's disease. Perlmutter Health Center, Naples, Florida, 239-649-7400. The glutathione solution can be sent anywhere and administered by a competent health-care practitioner.

Hyaluronic acid tablets. Reduces swelling and pain. Willner's Chemists, 800-633-1106.

Intense light. For insomnia, pain, and inflammation. Living Sunshine, ecoquest.com.

Ketogenic diet. For epilepsy. Complete information about this diet is in the book *The Ketogenic Diet: A Treatment for Children and Others* *with Epilepsy* by John Mark Freeman et al. (New York: Demos Medical Publishing, 2007).

Magnetic pads. Polar Power Magnets, 405-390-3499.

Ox bile. For digestion of fats and oils, especially helpful in gallbladder removal. Willner's Chemists, 800-633-1106.

Pregnenolone (natural). Dr. Ray Peat, Kenogen, P.O. Box 5764, Eugene, OR 97405, 541-345-9855; Willner's Chemists, 800-633-1106.

Progesterone (natural). Dr. Ray Peat, Kenogen, P.O. Box 5764, Eugene, OR 97405, 541-345-9855; Willner's Chemists, 800-633-1106.

NOTES

Introduction

1. Heather Pringle, *The Mummy Congress: Science, Obsession, and the Everlasting Dead* (New York: Hyperion, 2001).

Chapter 1

1. Sang Whang, *Reverse Aging* (Miami, FL: JSP Publishing, 1990).
2. *For Tomorrow's Children* (Blooming Glen, PA: Preconception Care, 1990).
3. Ray Peat, *Generative Energy* (Eugene, OR: self-published, 1994).
4. Keichi Morishita, *The Hidden Truth of Cancer* (Oroville, CA: George Ohsawa Macrobiotic Foundation, 1984).
5. Whang, *Reverse Aging.*
6. Malachy McCourt, *A Monk Swimming: A Memoir* (New York: Hyperion, 1998).

Chapter 2

1. R. A. Wiley, *Bio Balance* (Hurricane, UT: Essential Science Publishing, 1998).
2. Weston A. Price, *Nutrition and Physical Degeneration* (San Diego, CA: Price-Pottenger Nutrition, 2008).
3. Carol Goodstein, "Interview: Gary Nabhan," *Omni* 16, no. 10 (July 1994).
4. Roger Williams, *Nutrition Against Disease* (New York: Bantam Books, 1978).
5. Max Gerson, *A Cancer Therapy* (Bonita, CA: Gerson Institute, 1999).

6. Adapted from *Healthview* newsletter, November 1977.
7. Arthur F. Coca, *The Pulse Test* (New York: St. Martin's Press, 1994).
8. Ibid.
9. Nicholas Gonzalez, M.D., interview, *New Life*, March–April 2000, 31–35.
10. Thomas Cowan, "Raw Milk," *Price-Pottenger Journal of Health and Healing* 21, no. 2: 1, 4.
11. P. Khosla and K. C. Hayes, "Dietary trans-monounsaturated fatty acids negatively impact plasma lipids in humans: critical review of the evidence," *Journal of American College Nutrition* 15, no. 4 (August 1996): 325–39.
12. Udo Erasmus, *Fats That Heal, Fats That Kill* (Burnaby, BC: Alive Books, 1993).
13. "Breast Cancer and Dietary Fat: No Link Found," *New York Times*, March 10, 1996.
14. Erasmus, *Fats That Heal, Fats That Kill.*
15. Molly O'Neil, "Can Foie Aid the Heart? A French Scientist Says Yes," *New York Times*, sec. 1, November 17, 1991.
16. J. A. Karjalainen, "A Bovine Albumin Peptide as a Possible Trigger of Insulin-Dependent Diabetes Mellitus," *New England Journal of Medicine* 329, no. 17 (May 2000): 3218–35.
17. Peter Billac, *The Silent Killer* (Alvin, TX: Swan Publishing, 2000).
18. Judith A. DeCava, *The Real Truth About Vitamins and Antioxidants* (Columbus, GA: Brentwood Academic Press, 1996).
19. Ibid.

Chapter 3

1. Francis M. Pottenger Jr., "Hydrophilic Colloidal Diet," *Price-Pottenger Journal of Health and Healing* 21, no. 1.
2. Leslie Bonci, *The Association Guide to Better Digestion* (Hoboken, NJ: John Wiley & Sons Inc., 2003). (Sponsored by the American Dietetic Association.)
3. Bernard Jensen, *Foods That Heal* (Wayne, NJ: Avery Publishing Group, 1993).
4. The Staff of Prevention Magazine, *The Encyclopedia of Common Diseases* (Emmaus, PA: Rodale Press, 1976).
5. Jean Carper, *Food—Your Miracle Medicine* (New York: HarperCollins, 1993).

6. Garnett Cheney, "Anti-Peptic Ulcer Dietary Factor," *Journal of the American Dietetic Association* 3, no. 21 (1950): 230–50.
7. The Staff of Prevention Magazine, *The Encyclopedia of Common Diseases.*
8. Jon A. Kangas, K. Michael Schmidt, and George F. Solomon, "The Effects of Vitamin E on Rats with Ulcers," *American Journal of Clinical Nutrition*, September 1972, 24–27.
9. The Staff of Prevention Magazine, *The Encyclopedia of Common Diseases.*
10. Carper, *Food—Your Miracle Medicine.*
11. Lynn Payer, *Medicine and Culture* (New York: Henry Holt and Company, 1988).
12. The Staff of Prevention Magazine, *The Encyclopedia of Common Diseases.*
13. Michael Crichton, *Five Patients* (New York: Ballantine Books, 1989).
14. The Staff of Prevention Magazine, *The Encyclopedia of Common Diseases.*
15. Ibid.
16. Ronald L. Hoffman, *7 Weeks to a Settled Stomach* (New York: Pocket Publisher, 1991).

Chapter 4

1. Edward Howell, *Enzyme Nutrition* (Wayne, NJ: Avery Publishing Group, 1985).
2. E. F. Kohman, W. H. Eddy, Mary E. White, and N. H. Sanborn, "Comparative Experiments with Canned, Home Cooked, and Raw Food Diets," *Journal of Nutrition* 14, no. 1 (April 1977): 9–19.
3. Review of an article, "Diabetes Danger in a Taste of Chinese," *London Times*, April 8, 1992.
4. Shingo Kajimura, Patrick Seale, Kazuishi Kubota, Elaine Lunsford, John V. Frangioni, Steven P. Gygi, and Bruce M. Spiegelman, "Initiation of Myoblast to Brown Fat Switch by a PRDM 16-C/EBP-Beta Transcriptional Complex," *Nature* 460, no. 7259 (August 27, 2009): 1154–58.

Chapter 5

1. Stephen E. Langer and James F. Scheer, *Solved: The Riddle of Illness* (New York: McGraw-Hill, 1995).
2. Dr. Jonathan V. Wright, "When the Other Thyroid Results Come Back 'Normal.' This Test Can Tell Why You're Still Sick." *Nutrition & Healing* 16, no. 2 (April 2009): 3, 8.
3. Dr. Richard Cordaro, interviewed by the author in his office in Bronx, New York, October 12, 2009.
4. Ibid.
5. Langer and Scheer, *Solved*.
6. Ray Peat, *Progesterone in Orthomolecular Medicine* (Eugene, OR: self-published, 1993).

Chapter 6

1. Mark Herzberg and Maurice Meyer, "Periodontal Disease and Cardiovascular Disease" (presentation at a meeting of the American Association for the Advancement of Science in Philadelphia), reported in the *New York Times*, February 17, 1998.
2. Oxford University Press, foreword to *Health Research*, by Commission on Health Research for Development (New York: Oxford University Press, 1990).
3. Lawrence K. Altman, "Study Finds Heart Regenerates Cells," *New York Times*, June 7, 2001.
4. Karen Springen, Mary Hager, and Anne Underwood, "Attackers," *Newsweek*, August 11, 1997.
5. Paul M. Ridker, Nader Rifai, et al. "Comparison of C-Reactive Protein and Low Density Lipoprotein Cholesterol Levels in Prediction of First Cardiovascular Events," *New England Journal of Medicine* 347, no. 20 (November 14, 2002): 1557–65.
6. Dr. David Altshuler, "Genetic Loci Associated with C-Reactive Protein Levels: Risk of Coronary Heart Disease," *Journal of the American Medical Association* 302, no. 1 (July 2009): 37–48.
7. Ray Peat, *Mind and Tissue* (Eugene, OR: self-published, 1994).
8. Kilmer McCully, *The Homocysteine Revolution* (New York: McGraw-Hill, 1999).
9. Peggy van den Hoogen, Edith Feskens, Nico Nagelkerke, Alessandro Menotti, Aulikki Nissinen, and Daan Kromhout,

"The Relation Between Blood Pressure and Mortality Due to Coronary Heart Disease Among Men in Different Parts of the World," *New England Journal of Medicine* 342, no. 1 (January 6, 2000): 1–8.

Chapter 7

1. Barbara Loe Fisher, "Swine Flu Vaccine Should Not Be Given to Children" (lecture given at the International Public Conference on Vaccinations, July 22, 2009). Also Nicolas Janus, Launay-Vincent Vacher, Svetlana Karie, Elena Ledneva, and Gilbert Deray, "Vaccination and Chronic Kidney Disease," *Nephrology Dialysis Transplantation* 23, no. 3 (March 2008): 800–807.
2. M. Iguchi, T. Umekawa, Y. Ishikawa, et al. "Clinical Effects of Prophylactic Dietary Treatment on Renal Stones," *Journal of Urology* 144, no. 2 (August 1990): 229–32.
3. Ibid.

Chapter 8

1. Sandra Blakeslee, "New Way of Looking at Diseases of the Brain," *New York Times*, November 10, 1999.
2. Dana Mackenzie, "The Shape of Madness," *Discover*, January 2000, http://discovermagazine.com/2000/jan/featshape.
3. The Staff of Prevention Magazine, *The Encyclopedia of Common Diseases* (Emmaus, PA: Rodale Press, 1976).
4. J. McDonald Holmes, "Vitamin B_{12} Deficiency and Memory Loss," *British Medical Journal* 2, no. 4986 (July 28, 1956): 228.
5. Abram Hoffer, *Orthomolecular Treatment for Schizophrenia* (New York: McGraw-Hill, 1999).
6. Hans Selye, *The Stress of Life* (New York: McGraw-Hill, 1978).
7. Chris M. Reading, *Your Family Tree Connection* (New York: McGraw-Hill, 1988).
8. Felicia Drury Kliment, *Eat Right for Your Metabolism* (New York: McGraw-Hill, 2006), 12–17.
9. Study cited by Daniel Goleman in "Forget Money; Nothing Can Buy Happiness, Some Researchers Say," *New York Times*, July 16, 1996.
10. Dr. Jonathan Wright, "Breakthrough 'Pig' Formula Leads to Mental Health Miracle," *Nutrition & Healing* 15, no. 12 (February 2009): 1–5.

11. Miles Atkinson, *Archives of Otolaryngology* 75 (1962): 220, cited in The Staff of Prevention Magazine, *The Encyclopedia of Common Diseases.*

12. "An Upside to Migraines? Less Mental Decline Found," Patterns, *New York Times*, May 1, 2007.

13. Cited in David Perlmutter, "Parkinson's Disease—A Preventable Illness?" Dr. Perlmutter's iNutritionals, inutritionals.com/ healthy-living/neurodegenerative-conditions/parkinsons-disease/ parkinsons-disease.

14. Chris Gupta, "Six Weeks to Parkinson's Improvement with a Single Vitamin," adapted from Dr. Jonathan V. Wright's newsletter, *Nutrition & Healing* 13, no. 3 (May 11, 2004): 1–3, communicationagents.com/chris/2004/05/11/six_weeks_to_ parkinsons_improvement_with_a_single_vitamin.htm.

15. Muhammad Amir Khan and Lucia Berti, "Alzheimer's Disease Affects Progenitor Cells through Aberrant β-Catenin Signaling," *Journal of Neuroscience* 29, no. 40 (October 7, 2009): 12369–71.

16. Hugh Fudenberg. Speech delivered at NVIC International Vaccine Conference, Arlington, VA, September 1997.

17. Jonathan V. Wright, "Bio-Identical Hormones . . . to Beat the Odds of Developing Alzheimer's," *Nutrition & Healing* 13, no. 2 (March 2006): 1–3.

18. David J. Llewellyn, Kenneth M. Langa, and Iain A. Lang, "Serum 25-Hydroxyvitamin D Concentration and Cognitive Impairment," *Journal of Geriatrc Psychiatry and Neurology* 22, no. 3 (September 2009): 188–95.

19. Study cited by Bart De Strooper and James Woodgett in "Alzheimer's Disease: Mental Plaque Removal," *Nature* 423 (May 22, 2003): 392–93.

20. Jane E. Brody, "Vitamin E May Slow Age Damage in Rats," Personal Health, *New York Times*, May 28, 1996.

21. Mary Sano, Christopher Ernesto, Ronald G. Thomas, Melville R. Klauber, Kimberly Schafer, Michael Grundman, Peter Woodbury, et al. "A Controlled Trial of Selegiline, Alpha-Tocopherol, or Both as Treatment for Alzheimer's Disease," *The New England Journal of Medicine* 336, no. 17 (April 24, 1997): 1216–22.

22. Hal Huggins, "The Hidden Dangers of Dental Care," subject of a radio interview in Dallas, Texas.

23. Ray Peat, phone interview by the author, June 5, 2001.

Chapter 9

1. Robin Marantz Henig, "Asthma Kills," *New York Times*, sec. 6, March 28, 1993.
2. Cited in Jin Dai, Changshie Xie, and Andrew Churg, "Iron Loading Makes a Nonfibrogenic Model Air Pollutant Particle Fibrogenic in Rat Tracheal Explants," *Americal Journal of Respiratory Cell and Molecular Biology* 26, no. 6 (June 2002): 685–93.
3. Ellen Ruppel Shell, "Does Civilization Cause Asthma?" *The Atlantic Monthly* 285, no. 5 (May 2000): 90–100.
4. The Staff of Prevention Magazine, *The Encyclopedia of Common Diseases* (Emmaus, PA: Rodale Press, 1976).
5. Carole Ober, "Variation in the Interleukin 4-Receptor α Gene Confers Susceptibility to Asthma and Atopy in Ethically Diverse Populations," *American Journal of Human Genetics* 66, no. 2 (February 2000): 517–26.
6. C. Edward Burtis, *Nature's Miracle Medicine Chest* (New York: Arco Publishing, 1974).
7. Ibid.
8. The Staff of Prevention Magazine, *The Encyclopedia of Common Diseases*.
9. Donald J. Massaro, Gloria DeCarlo Massaro, and Pierre Chambon, eds., *Lung Development and Regeneration* (New York: Marcel Dekker Inc., 2004).
10. Carl Stough and Reece Stough, *Dr. Breath: The Story of Breathing Coordination* (New York: The Stough Institute, 1981).

Chapter 10

1. Michael A. Weiner, *Maximum Immunity* (New York: Pocket Books, 1987).
2. Jonathan V. Wright, "Even More All-Natural Tools for Fighting Arthritis Pain—and They Taste Great Too!" *Nutrition & Healing* 11, no. 11 (December 2004): 6.
3. Suzanne Somers, *Ageless* (New York: Random House, 2006).
4. "San Diego Clinic Immunological Center Clinical Study on Cetyl-myristoleate (CM8) vs. Arthritis," harrydiehl.com/research2.html.
5. Dr. Ludwig E. Blau, "Can Eating Cherries Cure Gout?" *Texas Reports on Biology and Medicine* 8, no. 3 (Fall 1950).
6. J. P. Seegmitten, *Gout* (New York: Grune & Stratton, 1967).

7. Dr. Jonathan V. Wright, "Osteoporosis Prevention Found in an Often Overlooked Hormone," *Nutrition & Healing* 14, no. 3 (May 2007): 1–4.

8. I. S. Klemes, *Industrial Medicine and Surgery*, June 1957, cited in The Staff of Prevention Magazine, *The Encyclopedia of Common Diseases* (Emmaus, PA: Rodale Press, 1976).

Chapter 11

1. Walter Pierpaoli and William Regelson, *The Melatonin Miracle* (New York: Pocket Books, 1995).

2. The Staff of Prevention Magazine, *The Encyclopedia of Common Diseases* (Emmaus, PA: Rodale Press, 1976).

3. Ray Peat, "The Transparency of Life: Cataracts as a Model of Age-Related Disease," *Ray Peat's Newsletter*, 1996, http://raypeat.com/articles/aging/transparency-cataracts.shtml.

4. Proceedings of the Symposium on the Biological Effects and Health Implications of Microwave Radiation, Richmond, VA, September 1969, cited in The Staff of Prevention Magazine, *The Encyclopedia of Common Diseases*.

5. Dr. Michele Virno, *Eye, Ear, Nose, and Throat Monthly*, cited in The Staff of Prevention Magazine, *The Encyclopedia of Common Diseases*.

6. Ray Peat, *Generative Energy* (Eugene, OR: self-published, 1994).

7. Gina Kolata, "After Cancer, the Health Problem That Most Frightens Americans Is Blindness," Science, *New York Times*, March 10, 1988.

8. Robert J. Rowen, "Reverse Macular Degeneration with a Single Doctor's Visit," *Second Opinion*, Spring 2008, 1–2.

9. Ibid.

Chapter 12

1. Gary Paul Nabhan, "About All You Can Eat: Feast or Famine," produced by the Scientific American Frontiers and sponsored by the GTE Corporation (Fall 1990–Spring 2000), pbs.org/safarchive/4_class/45_pguides/pguide_502/4552_feast.html.

2. Richard A. Passwater, *Lipoic Acid: The Metabolic Antioxidant* (New York: McGraw-Hill, 1995).

3. John Marion Ellis, "Diabetes New Therapies," *Price-Pottenger Journal of Health and Healing* 19, no. 3 (Fall 1995).

4. Passwater, *Lipoic Acid.*
5. Lester Packer, Eric H. Witt, and Hans Jürgen Tritschler, "Alpha-Lipoic Acid as a Biological Antioxidant," *Free Radical Biology and Medicine* 19, no. 2 (1995): 227–50.
6. Passwater, *Lipoic Acid.*
7. Denise Grady, "A Diabetes Treatment Fails to Live Up to Early Promise," Science Times, *New York Times*, September 28, 2006.
8. F. Bruder Stapleton, "Does Early Vitamin D Supplementation Prevent Type 1 Diabetes?" *Journal Watch Pediatrics and Adolescent Medicine*, April 23, 2008, http://pediatrics.jwatch.org/cgi/content/full/2008/423/1.

Chapter 13

1. Joyce Wolkomir and Richard Wolkomir, "When Bandogs Howl and Spirits Walk," *Smithsonian*, January 2000, 38–44.
2. Sara C. Mednick, *PNAS (Proceedings of the National Academy of Sciences)*, June 8, 2009.
3. Lucien Levy-Bruhl, *The "Soul" of the Primitive* (London: George Allen and Unwin Ltd., 1965).
4. Ray Peat, *Generative Energy* (Eugene, OR: self-published, 1994).

Chapter 14

1. Josie Glausiusz, "Homo Intoxicatus," *Discover*, June 2000, 20–25.
2. Roger Williams, *Nutrition Against Disease* (New York: Bantam Books, 1978).
3. Ibid.
4. Melissa Healy, "Study: Alcoholics Can Misread Faces," *The Seattle Times*, August 13, 2009.

Chapter 15

1. K. M. Pirke and P. Doerr, "Age-Related Changes in Free Plasma Testosterone, Dihydrotestosterone, and Oestradiol," *Acta Endocrinologica* (Copenhagen) 89 (1975): 171–78.
2. J. M. Holland and C. Lee, "Effects of Pituitary Grafts on Testosterone-Stimulated Growth of Rat Prostate," *Biology Reproduction* 22 (1980): 351–57.
3. Erik Ask-Upmark, "On New Treatment of Prostatitis," *Grana Palynologica*, cited in The Staff of Prevention Magazine, *The*

Encyclopedia of Common Diseases (Emmaus, PA: Rodale Press, 1976).

4. H. M. Feinblatt and J. C. Gant, "Palliative Treatment of Benign Prostate Hypertrophy: Value of Glycine, Alanine, and Glutamic Acid Combination," *Journal of the Maine Medical Association* 49, no. 3: 99–102.

5. "Benign Prostatic Hyperplasia (BPH)/Enlarged Prostate: Alternative Treatment," Urology Channel, November 2009, urologychannel.com/prostate/bph/treatment_alt.shtml.

6. Edward Giovannucci, Eric B. Rimm, Graham A. Colditz, Meir J. Stampfer, Alberto Ascherio, Chris C. Chute, Walter C. Willett, "A Prospective Study of Dietary Fat and Risk of Prostate Cancer," *Journal of the National Cancer Institute* 85, no. 19 (October 6, 1993): 157–79.

7. Demetrius Albanes, "Low Cholesterol Not Related to Prostate Cancer," *Cancer, Epidemiology, Biomarkers, & Prevention* 47, no. 8 (February 2009): 327–49.

Chapter 16

1. Study cited by Jonathan V. Wright in *New Secrets Every Woman Needs to Know* (Baltimore, MD: Agora Health, 2004).

2. Suzanne Somers, *Ageless* (New York: Random House, 2006). The author interviews Wiley.

3. "Interview with Dr. William Donald Kelley," *Healthview Newsletter* 1, no. 5 (1977).

4. Ross Trattler, *Better Health Through Natural Healing* (New York: McGraw-Hill, 1985).

5. Jane E. Brody, "Hormone Replacement Therapy: Weighing Risks and Benefits," *New York Times*, February 1, 2000.

6. Jonathan V. Wright, "How a Healthy Tan Can Decrease Your Breast Cancer Risk," *Nutrition & Healing* 14, no. 6 (August 2007): 1, 3.

7. Ibid.

8. T. S. Wiley, *Sex, Lies, and Menopause* (New York: Perennial Currents, 2004).

9. Ben C. Campbell and Peter T. Ellison, "Menstrual Variation in Salivary Progesterone Among Regularly Cycling Women," *Hormone Response* 37, no. 4–5 (1992): 132–36.

10. Ray Peat, *Generative Energy* (Eugene, OR: self-published, 1994).

11. William H. Parker, Michael S. Broder, and Eunice Chang, et al. "Ovarian Conservation at the Time of Hysterectomy and Long-Term Health Outcome in the Nurses' Health Study," *Obstetrics & Gynecology* 113, no. 5 (May 2009): 1027–37.

12. Mildred S. Seelig and H. Alexander Heggtveit, "Magnesium Interrelationships in Ischemic Heart Disease: A Review," *American Journal of Clinical Nutrition* 27 (1974): 59–79.

13. Stephanie L. Brown, Barbara L. Fredrickson, Michelle M. Wirth, et al. "Social Closeness Increases Salivary Progesterone in Humans," *Hormones and Behavior* 56, no. 1 (June 2009): 108–11.

14. Kristen Utheim Toverud and Guttord Toverud, "Studies on the Mineral Metabolism During Pregnancy and Lactation," *Norsk Mag. Laegevidenskap* 91, no. 53 (1932).

15. Sharon Begley, "Shaped by Life in the Womb," *Newsweek*, September 27, 1999.

16. Lawrence K. Altman, "High Level of Insulin Linked to Breast Cancer's Advance," *New York Times*, May 24, 2000. The study was carried out at Mount Sinai Hospital of the University of Toronto, and the findings were presented to the American Society of Clinical Oncology.

17. "Prevent Breast Cancer by Breast-Feeding," *New York Post*, January 31, 2001.

18. Nina Planck, "Death by Veganism," *New York Times*, May 2, 2007.

19. Sven Cnattingius, Lisa B. Signorello, Göran Annerén, et al. "Caffeine Intake and the Risk of First Trimester Spontaneous Abortion," *New England Journal of Medicine* 343, no. 25 (December 21, 2000): 1839–45.

20. Ray Peat, phone interview by the author, April 3, 1999.

BIBLIOGRAPHY

Aceves, J., and H. King. *Cultural Anthropology*. Morristown, NJ: General Learning Press, 1978.

Aihara, Herman. *Acid and Alkaline*. Oroville, CA: George Ohsawa Macrobiotic Foundation, 1986.

Anglesey, Debby. *Battling the MSG Myth*. Kennewick, WA: Front Porch Productions, 1997.

Bechamp, E. *The Blood and Its Third Anatomical Element*. London: John Ouseley Limited, 1912.

Billac, Pete. *The Silent Killer*. Alvin, TX: Swan Publishing, 1999.

Braverman, E., and C. Pfeiffer. *The Healing Nutrients Within*. New York: McGraw-Hill, 1987.

Carper, Jean. *Food—Your Miracle Medicine*. New York: HarperCollins Publishers, 1993.

Cawod, Frank. *Vitamin Side Effects Revealed*. Peachtree City, GA: Banta Company, 1986.

Coca, Arthur. *The Pulse Test*. New York: St. Martin's Press, 1994.

Colbin, Annemarie. *Food and Healing*. New York: Ballantine Books, 1996.

Crichton, Michael. *Five Patients*. New York: Ballantine Books, 1989.

D'Adamo, Peter. *Eat Right for Your Type*. New York: G. P. Putnam's Sons, 1996.

Erasmus, Udo. *Fats That Heal, Fats That Kill*. Burnaby, BC: Alive Books, 1993.

Fredericks, Carlton. *Psycho-Nutrition*. New York: Berkley Books, 1988.

Gerson, Max. *A Cancer Therapy*. Bonita, CA: Gerson Institute, 1999.

Hagglund, Howard. *BioBalance*. Hurricane, UT: Essential Science Publishing, 1989.

Hallman, Rick. *The Living Environment Biology*. New York: Amsco School Publications, 2000.

Hoffer, Abram. *Orthomolecular Treatment for Schizophrenia*. New York: McGraw-Hill, 1999.

Howell, Edward. *Enzyme Nutrition*. Wayne, NJ: Avery Publishing Group, 1985.

Kraus, David. *Modern Biology*. New York: Globe Book Company, 1995.

Langer, Stephen E., and James F. Scheer. *Solved: The Riddle of Illness*. New York: McGraw-Hill, 1984.

Matsen, John. *The Mysterious Cause of Illness*. Canfield, OH: Fischer Publishing Corporation, 1987.

McGarey, William A. *Edgar Cayce and the Palma Christi*. Virginia Beach, VA: Edgar Cayce Foundation, 1981.

Morrison, Marsh. *Research Report*. Cottage Grove, OR: Ecology Improvement Press, Inc., 1978.

Newbold, H. L. *Dr. Newbold's Type A/Type B Weight Loss Book*. New York: McGraw Hill, 1991.

Payer, Lynn. *Medicine and Culture*. New York: Henry Holt and Company, 1988.

Peat, Ray. *Generative Energy*. Eugene, OR: self-published, 1994.

———. *Mind and Tissue*. Eugene, OR: self-published, 1994.

———. *Nutrition for Women*. Eugene, OR: self-published, 1993.

———. *Progesterone in Orthomolecular Medicine*. Eugene, OR: self-published, 1993.

"Philippus Paracelsus." *Funk & Wagnalls*. New York: Standard Reference Works, 1967.

Philpott, William H. *Magnetic Health Enhancement*. Midwest City, OK: self-published, 1998.

Pierpaoli, Walter, and William Regelson. *The Melatonin Miracle*. New York: Pocket Books, 1995.

Randolph, Theron G., and Ralph W. Moss. *An Alternative Approach to Allergies*. New York: Harper-Collins Publishers, 1989.

Sahelian, Ray. *Melatonin*. Marina Del Ray, CA: Be Happier Press, 1995.

Schmidt, Michael A. *Smart Fats*. Berkeley, CA: Frog, Ltd. c/o North Atlantic Books, 1997.

Shute, Wilfrid E. *Vitamin E for Ailing and Healthy Hearts*. New York: Pyramid Books, 1974.

The Staff of Prevention Magazine. *The Encyclopedia of Common Diseases*. Emmaus, PA: Rodale Press, 1976.

Tips, Jack. *Your Liver . . . Your Lifeline*. Austin, TX: Apple-A-Day Press, 1998.

Trattler, Ross. *Better Health Through Natural Healing*. New York: McGraw-Hill, 1985.

Twentyman, Ralph. *The Science and Art of Healing*. Edinburgh: Floris Books, 1992.

Walker, N. *Become Younger*. Prescott, AZ: Norwalk Press, 1978.

———. *Fresh Vegetable and Fruit Juices*. Prescott, AZ: Norwalk Press, 1978.

Whang, Sang. *Reverse Aging*. Miami, FL: JSP Publishing, 1990.

Weiner, Michael. *Maximum Immunity*. New York: Pocket Books, 1987.

Williams, Roger. *Nutrition Against Disease*. New York: Bantam Books, 1978.

Wilson, Denis. *Wilson's Syndrome*. Orlando, FL: Cornerstone Publishing Company, 1996.

Wolcott, William. *The Metabolic Typing Diet*. New York: Doubleday, 2000.

INDEX

ABOUT THE AUTHOR

S tarting out as a teacher in the inner city, Felicia Drury Kliment was determined to find out what caused the learning disabilities and behavioral disorders in the children she taught. She found the answer when, as a faculty member at City College, she and a colleague conducted a research study that documented the adverse effects of processed food on schoolchildren.

This study, along with her own personal experience, consultations, and study of Chinese medicine and modern chemistry, caused her to come to the startling conclusions on which this book is based. Kliment's numerous articles on alternative medicine have been published in academic journals and popular magazines.